AF798316

The Fat Flush Plan

ADVANCE PRAISE FOR *THE FAT FLUSH PLAN*

"If you care about your life and state of health, this book will be a valuable resource for you."

— **Bernie Siegel, M.D.,** Author of *Love, Medicine & Miracles*

"Ann Louise Gittleman once again leads the crusade for better nutrition. She exposes the pervasive myths that all fats are bad and that unlimited carbohydrates are good. Sensible and thorough, her *Fat Flush Plan* is a terrific primer for anyone wanting to lose weight and regain vitality. We recommend it enthusiastically!"

— **Michael R. Eades, M.D. & Mary Dan Eades, M.D.,** Authors of *Protein Power*

"What a great program! Whether you're starting a diet with a bang or trying to budge the scales after a binge or just tuning up your body and hoping to lose some stubborn inches, this is a great, safe low-carb way to do it."

— **Fran McCullough**, Author of *The Low-Carb Cookbook*

"Weight loss programs are often long on claims and short on results. Ann Louise Gittleman's *Fat Flush Plan* offers great information and great strategies for weight management. A healthy, smart, safe, effective weight-loss program. What could be better?"

— **Tori Hudson, N.D.,** Professor, National College of Naturopathic Medicine and Author of *Women's Encyclopedia of Natural Medicine*

"In my Fit Camps, we work on lifestyle changes involving both nutrition and exercise. The Fat Flush Plan (Phase 1) has inspired my campers to initiate the dietary changes necessary for weight loss and better health."

— **Joanie Greggains,** Author of *Fit Happens*

"The Fat Flush is the healthiest and safest way I know to drop weight quickly. Ann Louise Gittleman has once again used her enormous talents and encyclopedic knowledge of nutrition and health to come up with a winning formula. Ann Louise has been one of the great influences on my professional life and one of the first people I turn to when I want a 'second opinion.'"

— **Jonny Bowden**, M.A., C.N., C.N.S. author of *Shape Up!*, the eight-week program to transform your body, your health, and your life

The Fat Flush Plan

ANN LOUISE GITTLEMAN,
M.S., C.N.S.

McGraw-Hill
New York / Chicago / San Francisco / Lisbon / London
Madrid / Mexico City / Milan / New Delhi / San Juan
Seoul / Singapore / Sydney / Toronto

Library of Congress Cataloging-in-Publication Data

Gittleman, Ann Louise.
The fat flush plan / Ann Louise Gittleman
p. cm.
Includes bibliographical references and index
ISBN 0-07-138383-2 (alk. paper)
1. Weight loss. 2. Reducing diets—Recipes. I. Title.

RM222.2 G5373 2002
613.2'5—dc21 2001052166

McGraw-Hill
A Division of The McGraw-Hill Companies

Copyright ©2002 by Ann Louise Gittleman. All rights reserved. Printed in the United States of America. Except as permitted under the United States Copyright Act of 1976, no part of this publication may be reproduced or distributed in any form or by any means, or stored in a data base or retrieval system, without the prior written permission of the publisher.

36 DOC/DOC 0 1 9 8 7 6

ISBN 0-07-138383-2

Book designed by Marsha Cohen, and set in Palatino by MM Design 2000, Inc.

Printed and bound by R. R. Donnelley.

This book is for educational purposes. It is not intended as a substitute for medical advice. Please consult a qualified health care professional for individual health and medical advice. Neither McGraw-Hill nor the author shall have any responsibility for any adverse effects arising directly or indirectly as a result of the information provided in this book.

Throughout this book, trademarked names are used. Rather than put a trademark symbol after every occurrence of a trademarked name, we use names in an editorial fashion only, and to the benefit of the trademark owner, with no intention of infringement of the trademark. Where such designations appear in this book, they have been printed with initial caps.

This book is printed on recycled, acid-free paper containing a minimum of 50% recycled de-inked fiber.

To my longtime agent and friend Mike Cohn —

Mike, this one's for you!

Contents

Foreword

There are three things in life that generate visceral responses: religion, politics, and nutrition. All three are often based on belief systems that do not respond well to challenge. In fact, those which challenge prevailing beliefs usually are ostracized because they question the orthodoxy no matter how wrong it appears to be. Of the three, nutrition is more of a science and therefore is governed by observation backed by experimentation.

My own journey in trying to make sense of the complexity of nutrition began twenty years ago when it became obvious to me that making fat the villain of nutrition was simply dead wrong. During the past twenty years, I have met many others who have shared my beliefs. One of the first was Ann Louise Gittleman.

I had known Ann Louise for more than twelve years when she first asked for my advice on fat-derived hormones called *eicosanoids* for her book entitled *Beyond Pritikin*. The two worlds from which Ann Louise and I came were totally different. I came from academia, whereas she was more of an observer of the outcome of standard nutritional advice. As the chief nutritionist at the Pritikin Institute, she was told that as much fat as possible should be removed from the diet. Although it seemed like an intuitively good idea, her observations at the Pritikin Institute made it very clear to her that many of the patients were becoming less healthy as they religiously removed fat from their diets. Sometimes the eyes tell us better than the brain.

Feeling that she could not in good conscience continue to recommend the Pritikin principles as the pathway to optimal health, she left to begin her own journey to understand exactly what we require for optimal health and then how to communicate the answer to others. Understanding why fat is essential to optimal health was the necessary first step, and then telling Americans that certain types of fat actually are good for them represented a far more difficult challenge.

This is why I find it interesting that Ann Louise's continuing journey, detailed in this book, has paralleled my own research. One of the key components of this new book is the role of certain fats, including fish oils, gamma-linolenic acid (GLA), and conjugated linoleic acid (CLA). All these have powerful effects on our hormones in general and in particular on the eicosanoids. In essence, these fats are powerful new "drugs" that we are just now beginning to understand how to use correctly. For the first time, it is correct to state it takes fat to burn fat.

The other key concept in this book is a term that most Americans hate to hear—it is called *calorie restriction.* However, this is now calorie restriction without hunger or deprivation. If you follow the recipes in this book, you will never be hungry or deprived, even though you are restricting your calories, because you are now controlling your hormones (insulin in particular) with laser-like precision. In the final analysis, what is going on in your body is incredibly complex, but how to orchestrate it is pretty easy as long as you are consistent and follow the basic dietary rules outlined by Ann Louise.

You also shouldn't be misled by the title, because this book is far more than simply a diet book. The only way to live a longer and better life is to control the hormones generated by the food we eat. Do we have all the answers yet? No, but this book represents a step in the right direction as we continually seek new information. Ann Louise's Fat Flush Plan is dietary common sense for all the right reasons—it is balanced, it is a program you can stay on safely for life, and it works.

BARRY SEARS, PH.D.
Author of *The Zone* and *The Anti-Aging Zone*

Preface

There are no quick fixes—but the Fat Flush Plan comes close. As a nutritionist always on the lookout to identify and correct metabolic and nutritional imbalance, I have searched beyond the conventional answers to uncover the root causes of unexplained weight gain. Thankfully, my investigative nature paid off. Years of hands-on experience and avidly following the latest research studies and diet trends led me to insights into lasting weight control.

The year 2000 marked not only the beginning of the new millennium, but also the birth of the expanded and complete Fat Flush Plan—a quick and easy way to erase those pockets of fat that bother us the most. That year was also when iVillage, the most popular women's health site on the Internet, approached me to be a guest expert on its Diet and Fitness channel. Honored to be a part of the leading Web site on women's issues, I introduced an early version of a diet plan called the Two-Week Fat Flush—the one I had used with my personal clients for fifteen years and which initially appeared as a brief chapter in my first book, *Beyond Pritikin*.

Suddenly people from every walk of life began to resonate to the concept of Fat Flush. In fact, Fat Flush received so many positive reviews within its first four months, along with over 400,000 hits monthly, that it soon became one of the leading traffic drivers of the Diet and Fitness channel.

The media picked it up and dubbed this initial diet blueprint the Internet Miracle Diet. Since then, the Fat Flush Message Board on iVillage has become one of the most popular diet and fitness boards in the history of the Web site—a fact which continues to amaze and intrigue me.

Magazines followed suit, featuring my rapid weight loss diet. *Woman's World* made Fat Flush its cover story in the early spring of 2000 as well as in January and February of 2001. *First for Women* also featured an adaptation of my diet on the cover, including my own testimonial and photo inside.

All of this unexpected national attention, however, did more than just spotlight this emerging diet plan. It was the catalyst for its development into a full-fledged book. The growing interest in my Fat Flush concepts—I had to post daily answers to mounting emails and conduct weekly chats just to keep up—generated a unique opportunity for me to hear directly from individuals all over the country.

In a very real sense, the invaluable iVillage community served as a focus group for me, providing significant input and helpful insights. The group also encouraged me to examine every aspect of the plan under a huge magnifying glass to learn why Fat Flush was supporting them on so many levels: body, mind, and spirit.

I soon realized that Fat Flush is more than a diet program. It is also a journey into self-care. As Jennifer Louden writes in the introduction of her book, *The Woman's Comfort Book*:

> Self-care is essential to survival, it is essential as the basis for healthy authentic relationships, it is essential if we honestly want to nurture the people we care about. Self-care is not selfish or self-indulgent. We cannot nurture others from a dry well. We need to take care of our own needs first, then we can give from our surplus, our abundance. When we nurture others from a place of fullness, we feel renewed instead of taken advantage of. And they feel renewed too, instead of guilty. We have something precious to give others when we have been comforting and caring for ourselves and building up self-love.

But that seems to be a difficult concept for many of us twenty-first-century women. According to a 1999 Wirthlin Women's Health Issues Survey, today's woman appears to be so entrenched in caring for the daily demands of work and family that she neglects the much-needed care of herself. Too often, she's penciled in at the bottom of her unending To-Do list. As a result, she falters under tremendous physical and emotional stress, totally drained of energy.

I believe that you deserve to put self-nurturing at the top of your To-Do list. That's why simple and healthy habits are built into the program, habits such as keeping a journal, moderate exercise, and going to sleep at a set bedtime. By following the total plan, you will not only enjoy effortless weight loss, but you will become renewed and revitalized.

As I heard from people across the nation, one thing rang loud and clear: They wanted more. Specifically, they asked for menu plans, recipes, a transition plan, a maintenance plan, and tips on how to follow the Fat Flush principles in a restaurant, how to Fat Flush during the holidays, and how to modify Fat Flush for men or women in different ages and stages of life (such as breastfeeding, pregnancy, perimenopause, or menopause). They also wanted to know how I developed the program, the science behind the protocol, and why each of the rather unusual elements was included, especially the flaxseed oil and the Fat Flush signature drink, the Long Life Cocktail.

Potential Fat Flushers asked to read testimonials, case histories, and success stories to reassure themselves and inspire them into action. Many had questions on how much to exercise and what kinds were appropriate. And it seemed as though everyone wanted to know what were the best fat-burning, brand-name supplements available to maximize their results.

I listened carefully to all the feedback, then decided to put it all together in a book. The three-phase *Fat Flush Plan* is committed to encouraging accelerated weight loss and ongoing, balanced weight control as well as championing lifestyle habits that are overlooked or forgotten as a result of our hectic day and age.

The first part of the book introduces you to the progression of the Fat Flush phenomenon and the five hidden weight-gain factors. You'll not only read the science behind each one, but you'll learn all about how each facet of the Fat Flush protocol addresses each factor. And I know you will feel encouraged by reading some of the inspiring testimonials, observations, and stories other Fat Flushers, like yourself, have sent me.

Then we move on to the easy Fat Flush game plan. You'll gain a practical understanding of the principles behind each phase of the plan and see how simple it is to put them into action as you graduate from one level to the next. There are details about the fat-burning supplements needed for each phase with helpful tips and words of wisdom from Fat Flushers who have been there. And you'll discover the power of ritual in your life in supporting your weight-loss goals. You'll learn how to keep a daily journal, tracking your progress, eating patterns, and emotional triggers. You will also discover how to sculpt a fat-resistant, cellulite-free body—without strenuous exercises. And you will see how to boost your body's immune system, physical repair, and even fat-burning while you experience the "art" of proper sleep and rest.

You will also find a wealth of information at your fingertips, including the Master Shopping List with name brands (like the best-tasting flaxseed oils) and quick tips on food preparation and storage as well as useful health tips. You will also have more than thirty quick and delicious recipes, as well as ideas on how to modify your favorite recipes and holiday delights the Fat Flush way. You'll learn smart, no-stress ways to take Fat Flush on the road, whether it's eating out at your favorite restaurant, a business luncheon, or that special occasion.

The last part of the book gives you straight answers to the more commonly asked questions, about the plan itself as well as special concerns. You'll also find a comprehensive Resources section of helpful products, educational resources, nutritional organizations, medical/nutrition centers, labs, and compounding pharmacies where you can go to get more information about the items or ideas mentioned in this book.

As you embark on your Fat Flush experience, I'd like you to keep a few things in mind. You are an individual and so is your rate of weight loss. Your body is unique, which means your weight-loss challenges are not necessarily like your best friend's or even other family members'. You will discover your own roadblocks and learn how to remove them, one step at a time, at your own pace.

I've tried to make the plan as easy as possible for this reason. You will start slowly and gradually make a couple of dietary and lifestyle changes, one at a time, even before you start. By easing into each progressive phase, you won't feel overwhelmed.

And take things one day at a time. Remember, Fat Flush is a journey toward your weight-loss destination. Be kind to and supportive of yourself. It's important to learn how to recognize and applaud even your smallest accomplishments of the day. And even if you slip sometimes—as we all do—that's okay. It's called being human.

Finally, know that you are not alone. I will be there with you to help guide the way because I also have been there. You and I will do this together. Be patient with yourself.

Let your journey begin . . .

ANN LOUISE GITTLEMAN

Acknowledgments

The behind the scenes story of the Fat Flush Plan is a book all by itself. There were many individuals who were instrumental and exceedingly helpful in making this book a reality.

My heartfelt thanks and appreciation go to fitness expert and KGO radio host Joanie Greggains, whose support throughout the years in the San Francisco Bay area has made Fat Flush a real sensation. Joanie's Fit Happens camps have successfully utilized the Fat Flush protocol with extraordinary results. I am also indebted to Joanie's outstanding assistant, Cindy Renshaw.

Mega thanks also to radio host Frankie Boyer of business 1060 AM WBIX for putting Boston on Fat Flush. And to Randy Featherston of KBJS 90.3 radio for putting East Texas on Fat Flush.

My thanks to Howard Schiffer, Adam Whizen, Ned Rosenthal, Jeannette Boudreau, and Richard Pine for their advice and suggestions in the early stages of my project.

My eternal gratitude to my editor, Nancy Hancock, for her professional savvy, marketing expertise, and diet know-how. Nancy has been in my corner for a long time, and this book finally gave us the opportunity to work together. I hope this will be the beginning of a long and mutually beneficial relationship.

I also am very appreciative of the efforts of the total McGraw-Hill team—including the publisher, Phillip Ruppel; the vice president of marketing, Lynda Luppino, and her staff, Lydia Rinaldi and Eileen Lamadore; the publicity director, Ann Pryor; and the editing and production team, Ruth Mannino, Clara Stanley, Paisley Strellis, and Michael Mendelsohn—whose enthusiasm and excitement contributed immeasurably to this project.

Thanks to my colleague and friend Zone guru, Dr. Barry Sears, for his pioneering genius, which ushered in a new era of nutrition.

Thanks to both Ann Castro and J. Lynne Dodson for their timely literary assistance.

Thanks also to my trusty assistant Krystie Gummer, who proved herself to be a top researcher as well as my responsible "right hand."

Stuart Gittleman, who handles all business aspects of ALG Inc., is to be acknowledged and thanked from the bottom of my heart for managing my calendar and schedule during the writing of this book. Stuart is simply *the* best, displaying dignity, grace under pressure, and an indelible sense of humor.

I would be very remiss if I did not thank my parents, Edith and Arthur Gittleman, who, for the summer of 2001, gave me back my old room, fed me three square Fat Flushing meals a day, and allowed me the use of their phones, fax, and email service so that I could do this book. We should all be blessed with such devoted parents. May they live till 120.

And thanks to my "significant other" TEX JWT for understanding and giving me his blessing to be back East to do this book!

My most sincere thanks to cyberspace angel Rose Grandy, her mother Ellen Buier, and her husband Christopher Grandy who were my taste testers and recipe mavens. Rose has become quite the Fat Flush expert and has been a gem to work with. Ditto for Monica Papoulias, whose assistance with my Fat Flush message board has been so very helpful.

A big hug to all the iVillage community members for making Fat Flush such a hit. Special thanks to Allison Rand and Emily Lapkin for always being there to update, revise, and assist with the messaging board.

David Filcoff, N.D., Arleen Barlow, and Linda Hooper kept me together—body, mind, and spirit—during the preparation of this manuscript, for which I am most grateful.

Thanks also to my wonderful friends who have supported this project wholeheartedly: Roy and Diane Speiser; Herb Shapiro; Paula Breen; Elizabeth and Monroe Krichman; Dick and Dianna Frederick; Helen and Bill Malm; John Coleman, Ph.D. and Lena Coleman; G. Green; Esterina and Shmuel Tafrizi; and the entire Paul Bindell family.

Last but not least, I thank you, my faithful readers, followers, and Internet visitors, whose letters, emails, and testimonials have motivated me to expand my Fat Flush vision into the plan. Blessings and besos to all.

CHAPTER

1 Someone Like You . . .

Every mighty oak was once a nut that stood its ground.

Weight gain, bloating, and those stubborn fat deposits on your hips, thighs, and buttocks—the very thought rattles your senses, not to mention your self-esteem. It's downright frustrating, to say the least. And believe me, you're not alone. There are more than 100 million of us currently fighting the infamous battle of the bulge. For most of us, it's a rigorous combat at best, trying one diet plan after another. Some regimens are too hard to follow, whereas others lack any real variety or satiety. In the end, we usually wind up back where we started—unhappy and overweight once again.

Over the years, I've had my own struggles with weight gain. Right from the start, I had to deal with a stacked deck, genetically speaking. Part of my body shape—the proverbial pear—I inherited from my mother and her side of the family, judging from the pictures of my maternal grandmother, aunts, and female cousins that graced our den wall when I was growing up. And like me, all the women on my mother's side were always on a diet, trying to lose those infamous last 10 to 20 pounds that seemed to stockpile below the waist.

On my father's side, my family history of diabetes didn't help matters any. From as early as I can remember in both junior high and high school, I suffered from low blood sugar, or "reactive hypoglycemia." I was always craving something sweet (such as cookies, candy, cake, or ice cream) to raise my blood sugar, which really piled on the pounds. I simply couldn't find the time to eat on schedule. Back then (much like today), I was too busy being responsible and a caretaker for everyone else—being a high school correspondent for the *Hartford Courant* newspaper, serving as the president of the Service Club, and teaching religious school after regular school—that I ignored my own body. So it's no wonder that I was always going up and down on the weight scale.

My use of food as an anesthetic to offset the stress of a competitive college environment during my freshman and sophomore years only compounded the matter. I would drift into one dorm for lunch and then into another one for yet another meal. In fact, men used to love to take me out because I didn't drink but had a hearty appetite. The truth is that I could eat anyone under the table. In addition, my body never seemed to firm up the way some women's do when they exercise. Moreover, I had to literally force myself to exercise anyway.

THE FAT FLUSH GENESIS

I spent my junior year abroad in London. There I started to frequent health food restaurants. Vegetarianism and drugless healing fascinated me. My whole life took an about-face once I began a program of cleansing and detoxification. (Which, by the way, helped me lose fat from those stubborn hips of mine rather effortlessly!) For the first time, I realized that whole foods, herbs, and dietary supplements could become a path not just to healing and wholeness but also to weight loss.

Back in the United States, after I graduated from college I decided to enroll in the New York Institute of Dietetics as part of the Dietetic Technician Program. Later, I received a master's degree in nutrition education from Teachers College at Columbia University. Later on, I became a certified nutrition specialist (C.N.S.) with accreditation from the American College of Nutrition.

It was a classroom experience at Columbia, however, that foreshadowed the nature of my professional journey and eventual Fat Flush discovery. While I was a student there, I heard the "Lamppost Story," which continues to this day to motivate me. It goes something like this:

> A gentleman goes out for a walk on an extremely dark evening and arrives at his destination, only to find that he has lost his wallet along the way. He immediately retraces his steps and starts looking for the wallet under the lamppost, where there is light. But he is unable to find his wallet because he had really lost it in the dark, where the light didn't reach. The moral of the story is that the answers are out there somewhere; you just have to look in the right places that have yet to come to light.

Inspired by this to search for answers beyond where the light was already shining, I was convinced that the real answers to weight gain, cellulite, and bloating were out there somewhere. I believed that we had yet to search in the right places, evidenced by the enormous amount of unsuccessful diet plans. Thus I embarked on a quest to find the missing links to weight loss. In my heart, I knew that the answer wouldn't be like any other diet plan. It had to be a program that addressed the underlying sources of weight gain and also embodied sound nutritional guidelines.

Today, while many women in their thirties, forties, and fifties are concerned about their changing shape, I've been able to keep my body pretty much fat-resistant for nearly three decades now. And that's despite my heredity. I found that once I had discovered an entirely new approach to managing my weight, it no longer mattered how the genetic cards were stacked.

That approach is my Fat Flush Plan—a program based on a unique diet model using healthful essential fats, balanced proteins, colorful carbohydrates, and a strict daily routine. It is designed to address and correct the most prevalent underlying causes of weight gain. These unseen causes have nothing to do with your genes. Instead, they reflect simple body chemistry imbalances that you probably never suspected. I call them the *five hidden weight gain factors*, which are the key to just about all of our overweight and obesity issues. You'll find that most diet plans typically target only one or two of these factors, which may explain why they don't work in the long term and cause recurring weight gain.

Ignored, overlooked, or simply not taken seriously enough, the five hidden weight gain factors include the following: an overworked liver, lack of fat-burning fats, too much insulin, the stress-fat cycle, and a unique take on "when fat is not fat." These factors are caused by a stagnant lymph system, sneaky food allergies, birth control pills, hormone-replacement therapy, and medications. You will learn all about these problematic factors in the next chapter, along with the scientific developments behind each factor that have reached a critical stage only in the past decade.

The discovery of my Fat Flush Plan didn't happen overnight. It progressed naturally out of every area of my life, from my personal weight control quest and working alongside my nutritional mentors to a wide variety of professional experiences spanning my entire career in counseling, consulting, and researching.

Early in my career, I had the privilege of working beside such nutritional pioneers as Hazel Parcells, Ph.D. and Nathan Pritikin. Their contributions helped me on my own weight control journey, which in turn enabled me to assist thousands of my own clients in their weight control efforts. In fact, when my first book, *Beyond Pritikin,* came out, my private practice in California grew, and soon people everywhere were resonating to my message that essential fats were absolutely necessary for rapid weight loss, longevity, and good health. For years I had a thriving practice that included sports figures, movie stars, fashion designers, producers, and members of the Joffrey Ballet. In this way, I was helping others who in turn were helping me fine-tune my program and stay on track myself as the messenger of a new weight loss approach.

Discovery: The Liver, Your Major Fat-Burning Organ, and the Lymph, Your Major Fat-Processing System

Over twenty-five years ago, a health-conscious friend shared an ad with me about the Parcells School of Scientific Nutrition in Albuquerque, New Mexico. The ad promised "five days that would change your life." Nothing could have been truer. After meeting Hazel Parcells, Ph.D., D.C., N.D., my life was changed forever. She inspired me to become a nutritionist with a foot in both clinical and holistic nutrition. Dr. Parcells was eighty-four years old when I met her—and lived to the incredible age of 106. A true pioneer in natural medicine, she was a woman ahead of her time.

Under Dr. Parcells' masterful tutelage, I first became acquainted with several innovative concepts, many of which later became the foundation of my Fat Flush Plan. The first revelation was the surprising connection between weight loss and the liver. I recognized early on what researchers are only now beginning to understand—that not only is the liver the main organ for detoxifying pollutants and chemicals in the body, but this vital organ also is a hidden key to effortless weight loss.

Based on simple biochemistry and the charts from *Gray's Anatomy,* I learned first hand that one of the best kept secrets to weight loss and lasting weight control is keeping the liver, the key organ for fat metabolism, in tip-top shape. For example, bile, which is synthesized and secreted by the liver and stored in the gallbladder, helps the liver break down fats. Bile cannot do its job, however, if it is lacking certain nutrients that make up the bile salts or if it is congested or thickened with chemicals, toxins, excess sex hormones, drugs, and/or heavy metals.

So I researched all the "liver loving" foods and nutrients that would enable the body to produce quality bile and aid in thinning it out. Since one of the primary ingredients of bile is lecithin—a highly effective emulsifier with a detergent-like ability to break up fats—I decided to experiment with adding lecithin-rich eggs to my daily diet. Soon, the addition of fresh lemon juice and water—a well-known bile thinner—followed suit twice a day. Not only did my own cholesterol come down (a good 20 points to be exact), but so did my weight.

Just to make sure I was onto something, I enrolled thirty of my clients in a six-week dietary exploration and instructed them to add at least two eggs daily to their current diet regimens and to add lemon juice and water twice a day—without changing anything else in terms of diet or exercise. Without exception, they all lost weight, especially around the waistline. In fact, one woman lost 21 pounds over the six-week period. I instructed the group to avoid caffeine and medications (including over-the-counter drugs) as much as possible because I suspected even then that these "drugs" were especially toxic to the liver.

Today, light is finally being shed on this vitally important organ. Many laboratories specializing in functional medicine testing offer a liver function test to determine how well the liver's two distinct detoxification pathways, the cytochrome P-450 phase I and phase II detoxification enzymes, are working. An individual ingests caffeine, Tylenol, and aspirin, and then specimens of saliva and urine are taken and analyzed to assess how well the liver is breaking down these substances.

The liver's two detoxification pathways are responsible for breaking down, eliminating, and neutralizing toxins. In this petrochemical world of ours, the sheer number of toxins we ingest from medications, drugs, pollutants, and pesticides can overwhelm the liver's ability to break them down and deactivate them. In addition, the detoxification pathways can become drained of the antioxidants, enzymes, and other nutrients necessary for detoxification because of the overload. The resulting metabolic by-products of incomplete detoxification are often more poisonous to the body than the original toxins.

The April 2001 *Consumer Reports on Health* provided an extremely helpful list of medications and herbs that can harm the liver with long-term use. The list included common medications (such as ibuprofen); cholesterol-lowering drugs (such as Lipitor); antidiabetic drugs; triglyceride-lowering drugs; anticonvulsants; estrogens used to treat menopausal symptoms (such as Premarin and Ogen) and those used in birth control pills (such as Lo/Ovral and Triphasal); and the herbs chaparral, comfrey, and pennyroyal.

The bottom line is that with so many toxins being dumped into the bile, its storage, concentration, production, and ability to digest fats are seriously impaired.

Another valuable insight I learned from Dr. Parcells was that cellulite—that dimpled accumulation of stored fat on our thighs and buttocks—was more connected to a sluggish lymphatic system than to poor muscle tone or weakened connective tissues. The lymphatic system, a relatively unknown secondary circulatory system underneath the skin, rids the body of toxic wastes, bacteria, heavy metals, dead cells, trapped protein, and fat globules. In essence, the lymphatic system is the garbage disposal of the body.

These concepts were so innovative back then that Dr. Parcells was the only one talking about them. After her ideas on the liver and the value of cleansing began to take root, researchers (for example, Sandra Cabot, M.D. in Australia) and American doctors (for example, Leo Galland, Kenneth Bock, and Elson Haas) started to write about them. Parcells would have been proud to know that in 2001—nearly five years after her death—a well-respected cardiologist from Philadelphia, Gerald M. Lemole, M.D. came out with a book called *The Healing Diet*, which links lymphatic system health with overall wellness.

Thanks to Dr. Parcells, I was given a head start in learning about the importance of cleansing both the liver and the lymphatic system for effective weight loss and cellulite control.

Discovery: The Role of Fat-Burning Fats

Another major piece of the weight loss puzzle fell into place during my tenure as director of nutrition at the Pritikin Longevity Center in Santa Monica, California. In the early 1980s, Pritikin diet was widely credited with being the model for the low-fat, high-carbohydrate diet prescription. At the center, as well as later in private practice, I found that many women following this type of program were complaining about distressful premenstrual syndrome (PMS) symptoms and other health ailments. I began to study their diet and health histories, hoping to find some underlying patterns.

For the most part, I found that they were loading up on unlimited fat-free complex carbohydrates such as pasta, bread, crackers, potatoes, corn, and beans. I discovered that the more they overate wheat-based carbohydrates (in particular, pasta, bread, cereal, and crackers), the more they craved them—and the more they seemed to become depressed. And these high amounts of grains were somehow contributing to their bloating—along with all that fat-free milk and yogurt they used with cereal. The unlimited use of fat-free but yeast-related seasonings such as soy sauce, tamari, tomato sauce, and oil-free vinegar dressings of every persuasion added insult to injury. Of course, the reason they were overusing these kinds of seasonings was that their zero-fat meals lacked any real flavor.

As it turned out, these same women were the ones complaining about retaining fluid, feeling tired and cold, and having allergies and recurring yeast infections, in addition to severe PMS. Therefore, I recommended a highly touted gamma-linolenic acid (GLA)–rich supplement known as *evening primrose oil*, used widely by European doctors for PMS-related problems. And this is when the unexpected happened. Besides eradicating their symptoms, these women also experienced a welcomed side benefit—weight loss!

The GLA fat-fighting connection. Although generations have used the evening primrose plant for its many medicinal and healing properties, the oil in the seeds—containing the powerful GLA—was making a splash in the weight loss arena. In fact, it was through research conducted by David Horrobin, M.D., at the University of Montreal, and M. A. Mir, M.D., a senior researcher and consultant physician at the Welsh National School of Medicine in Cardiff, Great Britain, that helped me realize how the right kind of fat stimulates the body's metabolic ability to burn fat. Their work demonstrated that evening primrose oil was most effective for those who were overweight by at least 10 percent. The key to this calorie-burning mechanism appeared to be the way the GLA-rich evening primrose oil worked via the prostaglandin pathways, a network of hormones that control virtually all body functions at the cellular level.

The GLA found in evening primrose oil mobilizes the metabolically active fat known as *brown adipose tissue* (BAT). This special form of fat, if available in sufficient amounts, can burn off extra calories and boost energy. BAT is a special insulating kind of fat found deep within the body that surrounds your vital organs such as the kidneys, heart, and adrenal glands. It cushions your spinal column as well as the neck and major thoracic blood vessels.

The series I prostaglandins created from GLA are believed to regulate many aspects of metabolism. GLA-induced prostaglandins regulate BAT by acting as a catalyst to either turn it on to trigger calorie burning or turn it off to trigger calorie conservation. Prostaglandins are also connected to a metabolic process referred to as *ATPase*. ATPase is also known as the sodium pump, a biochemical process necessary to keep the right amount of potassium inside cell walls and too much sodium out. GLA-rich substances such as evening primrose oil, by means of prostaglandin activity, control the sodium pump, which in turn revs up metabolism.

Based on mounting evidence that essential fatty acids are important to overall health—from studies that started to appear in such prestigious medical journals as the *New England Journal of Medicine* in the mid-1980s—I published my first book, *Beyond Pritikin*. Released in 1988, the book became a best-seller. It featured a chapter entitled "The Two-Week Fat Flush" that, as I look back, was really the origin of today's Fat Flush Plan. I inserted this program in my book as an antidote to the high-carbohydrate, high-grain-based, yeast-rich, fat-free diets of the era. It contained a one-day sample menu and touched on liver cleansing for more efficient fat metabolism. The diet featured the GLA supplements I had worked with in my private practice.

In 1996 I updated *Beyond Pritikin* and altered the Two-Week Fat Flush by replacing the safflower oil component with omega-3–rich flaxseed oil. Flaxseed oil works much like GLA but helps the body burn fat even more efficiently by increasing the production of a certain group of prostaglandins or eicosanoids, as they were called in the 1990s.

When *Beyond Pritikin* came out, my private practice in California grew, and soon people everywhere were resonating to my message that essential fats were absolutely necessary for rapid weight loss, longevity, and good health.

Discovery: Excess Insulin and Fat Storage

By the mid-1990s it was becoming increasingly clear to me that the public finally was ready to accept my finding that a low-fat diet isn't good for you because of the emergence of yet another piece of the weight loss puzzle: Fat-deprived, carbohydrate-stuffed individuals were realizing, due to the popularity of such books as *The Zone* (Regan, 1995) and *Dr. Atkin's New Diet Revolution* (Evans, 1992), that they were seriously jeopardizing their weight loss attempts because of the insulin factor. A fat-free diet, low in protein but high in carbohydrates (even the highly touted complex carbs) keeps insulin levels elevated, which promotes fat accumulation since insulin is a fat storage hormone.

Thankfully, insulin awareness has ushered in a brand new era of balanced nutrition and has legitimized the return of insulin-lowering fats and proteins to America's dining tables. The Fat Flush formula of healthy fats, lean proteins, and slow-acting (low-glycemic) carbohydrates is right on the low-insulin track.

Discovery: When Fat Is Not Fat and the Stress-Fat Hidden Factors

I learned about the remaining weight loss stumbling blocks through my most dependable sources—you (my readers) and clients. Time and time again I was finding that even when some of my clients were doing everything else right, they still couldn't lose weight. Thanks to the nutritional assessment questionnaire and food diary record sheets I had every client fill out, a pattern began to emerge. I discovered that many of those who were resistant to weight loss had a history of long-term use of birth control pills, hormone replacement therapy (HRT), antidepressants, and other medications as well as hidden food allergies. In Chapter 2 you will learn that this kind of weight gain is really not fat per se but rather severely waterlogged tissues masquerading as fat.

In addition, I noted from my clients' assessment forms that those who had the hardest time losing weight were also those who were the most stressed out. They were living on caffeine (from 2 to 4 cups daily), juggling home and career, definitely not getting enough rest (four to six hours daily), feeling "on edge" most of the time, and reporting an increase in food cravings and fat storage, particularly in the abdominal area. I suspected that the adrenal glands—our "fight or flight" glands that produce hormones in response to stress—were intimately connected to the stress-fat cycle. And I had a very strong hunch that I could disrupt this cycle with some simple changes in lifestyle habits.

So I honed the Fat Flush Plan to include stress-relieving protocols (such as exercise and journal keeping) that would zap the stress trigger and accelerate weight loss. Probably the most vigorous stress-busting dietary suggestion was to increase protein—at least 8 ounces or more of poultry, fish, or lean meat—because the body has higher protein needs when it is under stress. Just by adding another couple of ounces of protein to lunch and dinner, I had elated reports from clients who were dropping two dress sizes in two weeks—at last!

You may be asking, "What about other hidden weight gain factors like low thyroid or chronic dieting that throw the body into a metabolic slowdown?" I believe that these are also valid but secondary to the five hidden factors I have defined and outlined above.

DESTINATION: A NEW BODY AND A NEW YOU

In Chapter 2, I explain how hidden weight gain factors can sabotage your weight loss goals. It has been only in the last few years that my understanding of the scientific basis for the Fat Flush Plan has come together. For over a decade I have been collecting the latest studies, research, and books (which are referenced in the back of this book) that have helped to substantiate my Fat Flush discoveries.

Finally, there is an answer for someone like you, like me, like all of us.

CHAPTER

2 Five Hidden Weight Gain Factors

We learn wisdom from failure, much more than from success; we often discover what will do by finding what will not do and probably he who never made a mistake, never made a discovery.

—Samuel Smiles

QUICK QUIZ

Your struggles with weight are not the result of simply too much food and too little exercise. A myriad of unsuspected elements come into play. Before we look more closely at these, take this Quick Quiz to put your own lifestyle in focus.

	Yes	No
Do you drink caffeinated beverages daily?	____	____
Are you taking antidepressants or prescription or over-the-counter drugs?	____	____
Do you eat margarine or foods made with hydrogenated (solid or semisolid) fats?	____	____
Do you take birth control pills?	____	____
Are you on estrogen- or hormone-replacement therapy?	____	____
Did you take antibiotics two or more times during the past twelve months?	____	____
Do you avoid fat at all cost (e.g., by eating fat-free yogurt and fat-free cookies)?	____	____
Do you often crave sweets, bread, or other high-carbohydrate foods?	____	____
Do you eat pasta, potatoes, bread, or other carbohydrates two or more times daily?	____	____
Does at least one meal a day contain processed and/or packaged foods (e.g., frozen entrées or luncheon meats)?	____	____
Do you eat fewer than two servings of protein (e.g., meat, eggs, or fish) daily?	____	____

QUICK QUIZ *(Continued)*

	Yes	No
Do you drink fewer than eight 8-ounce glasses of water daily?	____	____
Do you regularly sleep fewer than 8 hours a night?	____	____
Do you lead a high-stress life?	____	____
Do you frequently skip a meal because you are "too busy to eat"?	____	____
Would you describe your lifestyle as sedentary?	____	____

If you answered "Yes" to even one of these questions, read on to learn how you may be unknowingly sabotaging your efforts at weight control and what you can do to make a difference.

If you are like most people, the Fat Flush Plan is not your first attempt at weight loss. You've exercised, counted calories, and cut out fat, then protein, and now even carbohydrates. Perhaps you lost weight; perhaps not. Chances are you've regained most, if not all, of the pounds.

For thousands of individuals, the Fat Flush Plan has been different. They've lost pounds and inches and kept them off. I believe this is so because the plan, unlike any other weight loss program, targets the five hidden factors mentioned in Chapter 1 that bring on unwanted pounds:

✓ Liver toxicity
✓ Waterlogged tissues
✓ Fear of eating fat
✓ Excess insulin
✓ Stress fat

How do these factors really affect your weight? Over the past several years, I have followed the research and, in some cases, the work of the nutritional pioneers who spearheaded these breakthroughs to answer this question. If you are like most of the Fat Flushers who have followed my work, when you understand some of the no-nonsense reasoning and the science behind the plan, you'll march confidently toward your ultimate success.

HIDDEN FACTOR #1: YOUR TIRED, TOXIC LIVER

Poets and songwriters may wax poetic about the heart, but your liver is by far the most versatile organ in your body and one of the most important. Weighing between 2.5 and 4 pounds in adults, the liver is the largest internal organ as well. Between 3 and 4 pints of blood flow through it *every minute.*

The Vital Liver

Researchers now estimate that the liver performs nearly 400 different jobs. It is the body's most important organ, functioning as a living filter to cleanse the system of toxins, metabolize proteins, control hormonal balance, and produce immune-boosting factors. Many of these functions are essential to your overall health, for example, the liver's synthesis of fibrinogen and other blood-clotting factors to protect you when you are injured. However, other liver functions have a direct bearing on your weight loss efforts, and these are the focus of the Fat Flush Plan.

A Fat-Burning Machine. Each day your liver produces about a quart of a yellowish green liquid called *bile* that emulsifies and absorbs fats in the small intestine. Bile contains water, bile acids and pigments, cholesterol, bilirubin, lipids, lecithin, potassium, sodium, and chloride. The liquid is stored near the liver in the gallbladder, from where it is transported to the intestine as needed during digestion.

Bile, as briefly discussed in Chapter 1, is the real key to the liver's ability to digest and assimilate fats. It can be hampered from doing its job because of a lack of bile nutrients, congestion, or even clogged bile ducts, which hamper bile flow and result in less bile production. If there is not enough bile produced, fat cannot be emulsified.

If you have a roll of fat at your waistline, you may have what is commonly called a "fatty liver." Your liver has stopped processing fat and begun storing it, for reasons I'll explain in a moment. Only when you bring your liver back to full function will you lose this fat.

An Efficient Metabolizer. The liver metabolizes not only fats but also carbohydrates and proteins for use in your body. The organ has a triple role in carbohydrate metabolism. First, it converts glucose, fructose, and galactose into glycogen, which it stores. Second, when your blood sugar level drops and no new carbohydrates are available, the liver converts stored glycogen into glucose and releases it into your bloodstream. Third, if your diet is regularly low in carbohydrates, the liver will convert fat or protein into glucose to maintain your blood sugar levels.

The liver converts amino acids from food into various proteins that may have a direct or indirect impact on your weight. Many proteins, for example, transport hormones through the bloodstream; as you've read, hormone balances are crucial to avoid water retention, bloating, and cravings, as well as other health problems. Proteins also help transport wastes, such as damaged cholesterol and used estrogen and insulin, to the liver for detoxification and elimination through the kidneys.

A Potent Detoxifier. Perhaps the liver's most important function, and the one that puts it at greatest risk for damage, is to detoxify the myriad toxins that assault our bodies daily. A *toxin* is any substance that irritates or creates harmful effects in the body. Some toxins, called *endotoxins,* are the natural by-products of body processes. For example, during protein metabolism, ammonia is formed, which the liver breaks down to urea to be excreted through the kidneys. Other toxins you consume by choice, such as alcohol, caffeine, and prescription drugs (more about these later). Still others are the thousands of toxic chemicals we breathe, consume, or touch in our environment: pesticides, car exhaust, secondhand smoke, chemical food additives, and indoor pollutants from paint, carpets, and cleaners, among others. Under ordinary circumstances, your body handles toxins by (1) neutralizing them, as antioxidants neutralize free radicals, (2) transforming them, as fat-soluble chemicals are transformed to water-soluble ones, and (3) eliminating them through urine, feces, sweat, mucus, and breath. Working with your lungs, skin, kidneys, and intestines, a healthy liver detoxifies many harmful substances and eliminates them without contaminating the bloodstream.

The detoxification process has two phases that should work in close synchronization. Phase 1 uses a group of enzymes to break apart the chemical bonds holding the toxins together. Known as *hydroxylation,* phase 1 makes some toxins more water soluble and temporarily more chemically active.

Phase 2, known as *conjugation,* attaches other enzymes to the chemically altered toxins, or intermediates. These enzymes complete the conversion of the intermediates, producing substances that are nontoxic, water-soluble, and easily excreted.

When the Liver Is Overloaded

Your liver is a workhorse that can even regenerate its own damaged cells. However, it is not invincible. When it lacks essential nutrients or when it is overwhelmed by toxins, it no longer performs as it should. Hormone imbalances may develop. Fat may accumulate in the liver and then just under the skin or in other organs. Toxins build up and get into your bloodstream. Among the signs of "toxic liver" are

- ✓ Weight gain, especially around the abdomen
- ✓ Cellulite
- ✓ Abdominal bloating
- ✓ Indigestion
- ✓ High blood pressure
- ✓ Elevated cholesterol
- ✓ Fatigue
- ✓ Mood swings
- ✓ Depression
- ✓ Skin rashes

When your liver is sluggish, every organ in your body is affected, and your weight loss efforts are blocked. Blood vessels enlarge, and blood flow becomes restricted. A toxic liver is unable to break down the adrenal hormone aldosterone, which accumulates to retain sodium (and water) and suppress potassium. This can raise your blood pressure. The liver fails to detoxify the components of estrogen (estrone and estradiol) for excretion, so symptoms of estrogen dominance arise. Unable to carry out its activities to control glucose, a toxic liver can lead to hypoglycemia, which can produce sugar cravings, weight gain, and *Candida* overgrowth. A toxic liver is unable to process toxins, enabling them to escape into your bloodstream and set off an immune response. With repeated assaults from escaped toxins, your immune system becomes overworked. Fluid accumulates, and you may develop one or more autoimmune diseases such as lupus or arthritis. A liver overloaded with pollutants and toxins cannot efficiently burn body fat, and thus will sabotage your weight loss efforts.

Liver Stressors

Probably nothing you do to control your weight is as important as keeping your liver healthy. This means avoiding as many of the damaging elements (like alcohol) as possible while embracing liver boosters. Among the lesser known compromisers of liver function are caffeine, sugar, trans fats, medications, and inadequate fiber.

Caffeine. In his landmark book, *Caffeine Blues*, researcher and nutritionist Stephen Cherniske, M.S., addresses a dozen critical organs and processes affected by caffeine. Right now, I'll focus on the liver, but I'll have more to say about caffeine later in this chapter.

When you drink a cup of coffee or can of cola, the caffeine is absorbed throughout your body. According to Cherniske, the liver must detoxify this caffeine without the aid of your kidneys. The kidneys attempt to excrete the caffeine molecules via the urinary tract, but they are reabsorbed into the bloodstream too fast. Thus, the liver must detoxify the caffeine alone.

Women are particularly vulnerable to the effects of caffeine. Research has shown that women detoxify caffeine more slowly than men. Studies comparing caffeine's effects on men and women found that women performed less well on cognitive tasks and rated themselves as more tired and disorganized than men did within one hour of a dose of caffeine. This may result not only from more caffeine remaining in a woman's body longer but also from hormonal interactions with caffeine. If a woman is also taking birth control pills, she will need about twice the average time to detoxify any caffeine she consumes.

You may be thinking, "I only drink one or two cups of coffee a day." However, you may be unknowingly consuming much more caffeine, from chocolate, cocoa, tea, some soft drinks, kola nut and guaraná root supplements, and a host of over-the-counter medications, including Excedrin, Anacin, Vanquish, Midol, Cope, Premens, Vivarin, NoDoz, and Dexatrim.

Sugar. Annually, Americans consume over 150 pounds of sweeteners and another 15 to 20 pounds of artificial sweeteners per person. Once again, you may not even know you're consuming sugar. Food producers don't use it just for sweetening. Sugar helps retain color in foods like catsup, gives a brown crust to breads and rolls, and adds body to soft drinks. Cigarettes, toothpaste, aspirin—even hairspray and postage stamps—contain sugar.

And sugar, a simple carbohydrate, comes in many forms, not all of which you may recognize in an ingredients list:

✓ Glucose
✓ Fructose
✓ Sucrose
✓ Maltose
✓ Lactose
✓ Raw sugar, brown sugar, powdered sugar
✓ Molasses, maple sugar, honey, corn syrup, high-fructose corn syrup
✓ Synthetic sugars: sorbitol, mannitol, and xylitol

In the process of being metabolized, these sugars rob your body of valuable nutrients; some of these, such as zinc, are essential for liver function. Sugar also inhibits your liver's production of enzymes needed in the detoxification process. Your liver must go into overdrive to convert the sugar into fats such as cholesterol and triglycerides. Unfortunately, once the liver has made this heroic effort, the fats may pile up in your liver and other organs or accumulate in the most typical fat storage areas of your body—thighs, buttocks, and abdomen.

Sugar is also a favorite food of *Candida,* a yeast that can overgrow and not only bring on bloating and water retention but also stress your liver. The yeast causes sugar to ferment and form acetaldehyde, a neurotoxin that increases ammonia levels in your bloodstream and can damage the liver. In addition, your liver must work overtime to detoxify the toxins produced by the fungal form of flourishing *Candida,* compromising the organ's fat-burning ability.

Trans Fats. As I indicated in Chapter 1, I introduced to the public the concept of adding the right fats back into the diet in 1988. I was labeled a "nutritional heretic" at the time, but the concept is definitely mainstream nearly fifteen years after I came out as an advocate of fat. Not just any fat, of course, but the essential fatty acids that have shown themselves to be both healthful and helpful in weight loss. I'll have more to say about the latest findings later in this chapter.

What I have been urging you to avoid for years are *trans fats,* also called *trans fatty acids.*

Trans fats are created when vegetable oils are hydrogenated. This process produces solid or semisolid fats widely used in commercial baked goods and other processed foods and in fast-food restaurants. By adding hydrogen and metals, under high heat, processors create a very stable oil but have altered the oil molecules. Trans fats impede your liver's ability to burn fat. They retard the conjugation phase of detoxification, increase fatty deposits within the liver, and thicken the bile, thus impeding bile flow through the bile ducts. You'll find trans fats in margarine (not butter), hydrogenated and partially hydrogenated vegetable oils, shortening, as well as in processed foods made with these ingredients. As a general rule, the softer or more fluid the oil, the fewer trans fats it contains.

Medications. As with food, the medications you take must be processed before they can be used by your body. Once again, your liver plays an important role. Some drugs, however, cause the liver to work harder. Hormone-replacement therapy, for example, causes the liver to make more clotting factors, and the organ must work harder to break down the drug's hormones. Other drugs may produce waste products that can accumulate in the liver. Acetaminophen, the active ingredient in the popular pain-reliever Tylenol, is one such drug. Studies by researchers at the University of Texas Southwestern Medical Center found that 38 percent of more than 300 cases of liver failure and 35 percent of 307 cases of severe liver injury were associated with excessive acetaminophen use.

Other drugs that can potentially harm your liver are

✓ Nonsteroidal anti-inflammatory drugs (NSAIDs)
✓ Cholesterol-lowering drugs
✓ Antidiabetic drugs
✓ Triglyceride-lowering drugs
✓ Anticonvulsants
✓ Hormones (e.g., estrogen and tamoxifen)

In addition, to protect your liver, you may want to avoid these nutritional supplements, which when taken on a regular basis may actually damage it:

✓ Chaparral
✓ Comfrey
✓ Germander
✓ Pennyroyal
✓ High-dose vitamin A
✓ Anabolic steroids
✓ Ephedra *(ma huang)*
✓ Gentian
✓ Senna
✓ Shark cartilage
✓ Scutellaria (skull cap)
✓ Valerian

If you are currently taking any medications and have concerns about their effects on your liver, *do not stop taking the drugs before you consult your physician.* Liver function tests are available. You may be able to take an alternative drug with less potential for liver damage. Many drugs, for example, are available in lower doses or in different forms (e.g., patch, pill, or injection), or a natural form may replace a synthetic product. These alternatives may provide the treatment you need without the added weight and liver dysfunction you don't need. Know and weigh the benefits of the medication versus weight gain and any other side effects you're experiencing.

Inadequate Fiber. If you are like most Americans, you eat only about 10 to 12 grams of fiber a day when experts believe that 20 to 35 grams are ideal for long-term health.

Among fiber's healthful benefits is its role in moving toxins out of your body. Insoluble fibers, from flaxseed, for example, absorb water in your digestive tract. This speeds up transit time (the time it takes materials to move through your intestine) to move waste products out of your body. Without adequate fiber, up to 90 percent of cholesterol and bile acids will be reabsorbed and recirculated to the liver. This taxes your liver and reduces its fat-burning abilities. No matter what the cause, a sluggish, overworked liver does a poor job metabolizing fat, and you gain weight.

What the Fat Flush Plan Does for Your Tired, Toxic Liver

We start with the plan's cranberry juice–water mixture and Long Life Cocktail of cranberry juice, water, and psyllium or flaxseed as a potent source of phytonutrients such as anthocyanins, catechins, luteins, and quercetin. These powerful phytonutrients act as antioxidants, providing nutritional support and cofactors for the liver's cytochrome P-450 phase I and phase II detoxification pathways. These nutrients also seem to digest fatty globules in the lymph. The cocktail's fiber blocks the absorption of fat, increases fat excretion, and binds toxins so that they are not reabsorbed into your body.

The lemon found in the plan's hot water–lemon drink benefits bile formation, which is essential for optimal fat metabolism and helps regenerate the liver. It also promotes peristalsis, the movement in the bowels that keeps waste moving along the digestive tract and out of the body for elimination.

The plan's cranberry juice–water mixture and plain water will assist your liver in diluting and expelling the increased body wastes from the two-phase detoxification process. Water helps empty stubborn fat stores because your liver is more efficient at using stored fat for energy when your body is well hydrated.

Daily protein is important to your liver's health and function. Only protein can raise metabolism by 25 percent and activate the production of enzymes needed during detoxification to break down toxins into water-soluble substances for excretion. Your liver needs protein to produce the bile that is essential for absorbing fat-soluble nutrients. Protein also provides amino acids, such as cysteine, that your body needs to produce the antioxidant glutathione. This enzyme is one of several that overcome the damaging free radicals produced in your liver (and elsewhere) during detoxification.

Red meats such as lean beef and lamb are high in L-carnitine, which plays a vital role in normalizing liver enzymes in the blood and in the liver's use and metabolism of fatty acids. L-Carnitine, which is made primarily in the liver, is a cousin of amino acids and similar to vitamin B. This nutrient carries fat to the mitochondria in your cells, where the fat is converted to energy. L-Carnitine also helps clear waste products from the mitochondria to avoid free-radical accumulation (and damage) as a by-product of food oxidation. In animal studies, carnitine has been shown to protect the liver from powerful toxins. To ensure that you get enough of this fat-burning nutrient, the plan includes not only dietary sources but also a supplement. You'll get 1 gram or more of L-carnitine per day, which at least one study has shown is enough to burn off 10 extra pounds in twelve weeks when combined with a Fat Flush–type diet and light exercise.

By including flaxseed oil, the plan takes advantage of its metabolism-raising action and its ability to attract and bind to the oil-soluble poisons that lodge in the liver and carry them out of the system for elimination. The essential fatty acids in flaxseed oil also stimulate bile production, which is crucial to the breakdown of fats.

Eggs are the highest dietary source of several sulfur-based amino acids, including taurine, cysteine, and methionine. These are needed by the liver to regulate bile production. This nutrient-rich food is also a superb source of phosphatidylcholine, a nutrient needed for overall liver health and to make lecithin, which helps prevent cholesterol oxidation harmful to the liver and other organs. If you're worried about eggs and heart disease, take note: A dietary analysis published in *JAMA (Journal of the American Medical Association)* in 1999 followed nearly 40,000 men and 80,000 women over a period of eight to fourteen years. The study found no evidence of any association between egg consumption and the risk of coronary heart disease or stroke in healthy men or women. So enjoy up to two eggs a day on the plan.

You'll find lots of cruciferous vegetables in the menus. Broccoli, brussels sprouts, and kale are very high in sulforaphane, a substance your liver uses in converting toxins into nontoxic waste for elimination.

Many of the herbs and spices featured in the Fat Flush Plan were selected for their liver-supporting and fat-metabolizing properties. Garlic and onion encourage bile secretion and aid liver function. Gingerroot boosts metabolism, helps reduce toxin buildup in fat cells, and supports bile flow.

Supplements are an integral part of the plan, including the lipotropic herbs dandelion root, milk thistle, turmeric, and oregon grape root. Lipotropic substances decrease the fat storage rate in liver cells and accelerate fat metabolism. Dandelion root, which contains high levels of vitamin A and other nutrients, has been shown to aid the liver and fat metabolism in two ways. It stimulates the liver to produce more bile to send to the gallbladder while at the same time causing the gallbladder to contract and release its stored bile, thus assisting in fat metabolism.

Milk thistle, in use for over 2000 years, increases liver enzyme production, helps repair damaged liver tissue, and blocks the effects of some toxins. Over 100 research reports have been published on the liver-supporting properties of its active ingredient, silymarin.

Turmeric, a relative of gingerroot, is the highest known source of beta-carotene, one of the powerful antioxidants that help protect the liver from damage by free radicals. Oregon grape root helps stimulate the liver by helping to control bile production.

Among the other lipotropic factors featured in the plan's supplements are the B-complex vitamins phosphatidylcholine and inositol, the amino acid methionine, and the fat-digesting enzyme lipase. They help prevent excess fat buildup and thin or emulsify fat for easy movement through the bloodstream.

Just as important as what is included is what is excluded. Among the missing are caffeine; sugar; alcohol; yeast-based foods such as bread, soy sauce; most vinegars (except the anti-*Candida* apple cider vinegar); and trans fats from fried foods, margarine, vegetable shortenings, and commercial vegetable oils. These seriously disrupt liver function by clogging the detoxification pathways or increasing *Candida* production. The yeast-related poison acetaldehyde is extremely toxic to the liver and inhibits fat burning.

You also won't find several herbs popularized recently for their thermogenic qualities. Most widely known is ephedra, or *ma huang.* Ephedra acts as a stimulant to the adrenal glands, which are responsible for your body's stress response and for maintaining blood sugar levels. Prolonged use of ephedra can create adrenal exhaustion. The herb also can constrict blood vessels, elevate blood pressure, and raise the heart rate. These can be serious side effects, especially for individuals with diabetes, heart disease, hypertension, or kidney disease. Kola nut, guaraná, and mate contain caffeine, and the fifth thermogenic, white willow bark (from which aspirin is derived), is high in salicylate, which can have unwanted blood-thinning effects.

HIDDEN FACTOR #2: WHEN FAT IS NOT FAT

On a "good" day, your body is 60 to 70 percent water by weight. About two-thirds of the water is in your cells; the rest is in blood, body fluids, and spaces between cells. This water is essential. It flushes toxins, moistens your respiratory system, and is part of every metabolic process. Cells take the water they need from capillaries, which in turn carry waste products and excess water to the kidneys.

However, many individuals carry an extra 10 to 15 pounds of water trapped in their tissues. This water contributes to abdominal bloating, cellulite, and face and eye puffiness. It is what my esteemed colleague Elson

Haas, M.D., calls "false fat." That is, the weight is not the result of additional adipose tissue, or true fat, but of excess water. Waterlogged tissues result from various causes, including

- ✓ Consuming too little water and protein
- ✓ Food sensitivities
- ✓ Hormonal fluctuations
- ✓ Certain medications

Deficiencies and Water Retention

It's ironic, but consuming too little water can cause your body to retain water. Your kidneys must have adequate water to flush waste from your body. When your fluid intake is low, the kidneys hoard water.

Insufficient fluid also slows the lymphatic system. This system of organs, tissues, and tiny channels filters cellular waste and other foreign particles, pushing this debris along in lymph the contraction of the lymph vessels. Some researchers conjecture that when a sluggish lymphatic system fails to carry wastes away in a timely fashion, the waste accumulates in fat cells and causes cellulite. At least one study, conducted at Brussels University in Belgium and cited by Elisabeth Dancey, M.D. in *The Cellulite Solution,* has found that women with cellulite showed lymphatic system deficiencies.

Our obsession with protein and fat has abolished these nutrients from our diets and may contribute to widespread water retention. Protein plays a crucial role in tissue growth and healing, strengthening the immune system, and burning fat. But it is its hydrophilic—literally, "water loving"—properties that have an impact on water retention. Proteins that circulate in your blood control water levels between and within cells and within your arteries and veins by attracting water molecules. As the blood circulates through your kidneys, this excess water is removed and eliminated. When your body is deficient in protein, however, fluid leaks from the vascular spaces into the spaces between the cells. It becomes trapped there, resulting in cellulite, water retention, bloating, and water weight gain.

When You React to Food

An estimated 60 to 80 percent of people are sensitive to one or more foods. Unlike true allergies, sensitivities often cause delayed, rather than immediate, reactions after you eat the offending food. This delay can make it difficult for you to tie your symptoms to the food you eat. Among the vast array of food sensitivity symptoms are

- ✓ Headache
- ✓ Coughing
- ✓ Blurred vision

✓ Rapid heartbeat
✓ Indigestion
✓ Skin rashes
✓ Fatigue
✓ Joint swelling
✓ Mood swings

Food sensitivities are also one of the most common causes of weight gain through fluid retention and through overeating brought on by cravings.

The Response to Reactive Foods. Your body's immune system releases antibodies in response to signals from foreign substances. In the case of food sensitivities, the antibody is immunoglobulin G (IgG), found only in the bloodstream. The "foreign substance" is food macromolecules that have left the digestive tract and entered the bloodstream. When IgG meets a macromolecule, the entire immune response is kicked off. Histamines and other chemicals are released, and the area is flooded with extra fluid to wash away the reactive food particle. Your body holds onto this water as long as such molecules remain in your tissues.

At the same time, your body produces hormones, including cortisol and aldosterone, which increase sodium intake. This sodium attracts more water to the cells and tissues. In your gastrointestinal system, reactive foods can stimulate production of the gut hormones cholecystokinin and somatostatin, which cause water retention in gut tissues.

The production of histamine and other chemicals causes blood vessels to expand and contract, leaking fluids into tissues and setting off a secondary inflammatory response and swelling. This leaking fluid often carries protein with it, and the protein attracts sodium and still more fluid.

To compound the weight gain from waterlogged tissues, food sensitivities also trigger weight gain from adipose tissue. This results from either heightened cravings for reactive foods or disruption of your metabolism.

The same immune response that pumps excess fluid into your tissues also triggers your body's distress mechanisms, centered around various natural chemicals and hormones. First, endorphins hit your system. These natural opiates give you a pleasant feeling of relief—but only for a few minutes to several hours. As your supply of endorphins dwindles, you are uncomfortable and seek to recreate the pleasant feelings with more of the reactive food. Cravings strike!

Second, your adrenal glands release epinephrine, norepinephrine, and cortisol, which give you a burst of energy and a mood lift. When these hormones are depleted, fatigue and irritability set in. Once again, you crave the reactive food to bring back your energy level.

Third, your insulin levels become destabilized, which lowers your blood sugar levels. Cells are starved for this energy booster, and you are weak and starved for food, especially carbohydrates.

Finally, as if all this weren't enough, your levels of the neurotransmitter serotonin drop. This chemical is produced by the hypothalamus, the part of the brain that controls hunger, and is carried primarily by white blood cells. When you eat nonreactive foods, serotonin helps signal that you are full and shuts off your hunger. However, when your immune system goes into high gear in response to a reactive food, your white blood cells are too busy fighting the "invader food" to carry serotonin. The result is a craving for high-carbohydrate foods to help move serotonin to the brain.

Not surprisingly, these disruptions in hormone and chemical levels severely affect your metabolism and make putting on pounds oh so easy. Metabolism is slowed when your epinephrine levels are depleted, causing increased fat storage, or when your thyroid gland doesn't function properly because signal hormones are imbalanced. The thyroid gland is a key component of your body's fat-burning process. Some food reactions also interfere with your body's ability to absorb the fat-burning essential fatty acids—such as the GLA I mentioned in Chapter 1.

Food Triggers. What foods are most likely to trigger this destructive immune response? Elson Haas, M.D., Jacqueline Crohn, M.D., and others have identified the most commonly reactive foods. Among them are

✓ Dairy products
✓ Wheat
✓ Sugar
✓ Yeast

These account for up to 80 percent of food reactions, although almost any food can be reactive.

Reactions to these foods develop primarily because of poor digestion, which results in partially digested food macromolecules entering the bloodstream and setting off the immune response. Reasons for poor digestion vary from eating too fast to eating too little fiber to eating the same foods repeatedly. Excessive consumption of processed foods, loaded with corn syrup, monosodium glutamate (MSG), and gluten, is particularly disastrous. According to a 1996 report published in *Gastroenterology,* 1 in 250 people has a severe reaction to gluten, a protein-containing substance found in grain, such as wheat, rye, oats, and barley, that gives dough its elasticity. Gluten sensitivity arises most commonly with wheat, used in practically everything from breads and pastas to piecrust, muffins, bagels, and cakes. Gluten can damage the intestinal lining, create inflammation, and disrupt nutrient absorption, especially of the precious B vitamins. Consequently, if gluten-containing foods are your triggers, you may experience not only bloating but also eczema, fatigue, intestinal gas, and anemia.

Candida and Food Reactions: It's Overgrowth, Not Overweight. Among the most common reasons food enters the bloodstream before it's fully digested is candidiasis, an overgrowth of the naturally occurring yeast *Candida albicans. Candida* normally lives alongside millions of bacteria in your gastrointestinal tract, on your skin, and in your mucosa, esophagus, and small intestine. Your healthy immune system and these "helpful" bacteria keep the yeast in balance.

However, when your immune system is weakened, *Candida* can get out of control. It changes from a noninvasive spore form into a fungal form that grows thread-like mycelia. These structures bore through your intestinal lining, penetrate other cells, and extract nutrients. The *Candida* migrates to other tissues, producing toxins such as acetaldehyde that stress the immune system. *Candida* also produces hormone-like substances that interfere with normal hormone production. For example, it may stimulate increased estrogen production and interfere with hormone signals to the immune system.

The holes in your intestine allow food macromolecules to enter the bloodstream—the trigger for food reactions. Studies in rats have found that *Candida* also stimulates histamine production, another trigger in the classic allergic reaction. An estimated 80 percent of people with multiple allergies have *Candida* overgrowth.

Many of the symptoms of candidiasis mimic those of food reactions: fatigue, headaches, bloating, nasal congestion, heartburn, and moodiness, among others.

The relationship between candidiasis and food sensitivities is made even stronger by consumption of sugars and refined carbohydrates. The foods you are most likely to crave as a result of food allergies are the ones most enjoyed by the *Candida* cells—those sweets, chips, and pasta help create an environment that encourages yeast growth. This is compounded if you often consume food with a high yeast or mold content, such as dried fruit, bread, and beer.

A diet deficient in essential fatty acids, vitamins, and essential amino acids weakens your immune system and also can lead to candidiasis. In addition, *Candida* overgrowth commonly develops in women taking birth control pills or in anyone taking antibiotics or cortisone-type medications.

A Woman's Hormones: Natural and Synthetic

From puberty, women's bodies are subject to the effects of estrogen-progesterone balance. At ovulation, estrogen secretion increases fat production by inhibiting thermogenesis (fat burning). In turn, fat stimulates more estrogen production, which gives you more fat. At the same time, progesterone levels decrease, which is thought to stimulate production of anti-diuretic hormone with resulting water retention. This balance is a crucial component in your body's preparation for pregnancy, which requires increased body fluids and fat.

When Balance Is Lost. For too many women, however, this natural cycle is disrupted, and weight gain—from both actual fat and water retention—becomes permanent. Estrogen levels remain high, resulting in a condition known as *estrogen dominance.* Among the symptoms of estrogen dominance are fat gain (especially around your abdomen, hips, and thighs), sluggish metabolism, bloating, and water retention. Estrogen can promote sodium retention (and thereby more water retention). The hormone changes the way your body metabolizes the amino acid tryptophan, which is necessary to produce serotonin. You'll remember that serotonin deficiency can lead to food cravings and weight gain. When estrogen is much higher than progesterone, you may develop hypothyroidism. A healthy thyroid gland secretes hormones that help signal the pancreas to produce insulin. With a sluggish thyroid, your body may produce too little insulin and trigger low blood sugar (hypoglycemia), along with intense cravings for carbohydrates.

Fluctuating estrogen levels are only one-half of the equation, of course. Thanks to the pioneering research of Raymond Peat, Ph.D., and John Lee, we are becoming better informed about the role of progesterone. This hormone signals the hypothalamus to increase your core body temperature, thereby increasing your resting metabolism rate. Low levels of progesterone cause your body to burn 15,000 to 20,000 *fewer* calories per year and increase water retention. You may not produce enough because (1) you are deficient in zinc and vitamin B_6, nutrient precursors of progesterone, (2) you are not ovulating regularly, leaving you without a corpus luteum to create progesterone, or (3) your body is converting progesterone into other chemicals as a result of excessive stress.

High levels of progesterone, on the other hand, increase your appetite. They also slow down intestinal transit time to increase food absorption, which can increase insulin levels. The resulting additional blood glucose is absorbed by fat cells to add pounds of true fat.

Causes of Imbalance. Estrogen-replacement therapy (ERT) and hormone-replacement therapy (HRT) are common causes of estrogen-progesterone imbalances, with millions of American women currently on HRT. Research into the effects of these therapies on weight has found conflicting results. For example, when researchers gave monkeys estrogen with synthetic progestin (a form of progesterone), their weight increased, fat tended to accumulate around their abdomens, and they secreted excess insulin. On the other hand, monkeys given estrogen with natural progesterone did not experience these effects.

Several major studies with large groups of women have attempted to define the positive and negative effects of ERT/HRT, including weight gain and fat distribution. The Postmenopausal Estrogen and Progestin Intervention (PEPI) trial, reported in 1997 in the *Journal of Clinical Endocrinology and Metabolism,* found that over the study's three-year period, the women studied gained an average of 1.5 to 2.9 pounds, depending on the type of therapy given. Women taking part but receiving only a placebo (sugar pill) gained an average of 4.6 pounds.

If you are among the millions of women taking birth control pills to prevent pregnancy, regulate your menstrual cycle, or treat acne, an unwanted side effect may be weight gain. Contraceptives can create a state of anovulation, and the absence of ovulation can lead to progesterone deficiency, slowing metabolism and encouraging water retention. Birth control pills also aggravate problems with insulin regulation and resulting carbohydrate cravings, as well as encourage candidiasis.

Medication Bloat

Unfortunately, birth control pills and ERT/HRT are not the only medications that cause water retention, bloating, and weight gain. Chances are that your medicine cabinet contains one or more other prescription drugs that are undermining your weight loss efforts. Some antidepressants, for example, cause weight gain in 89 percent of patients taking them. Other types of drugs known to cause weight gain in some patients include

- ✓ Antiestrogens
- ✓ Antihistamines
- ✓ Beta-blockers and other blood pressure medications
- ✓ Corticosteroids
- ✓ Diabetes medications
- ✓ Nonsteroidal anti-inflammatory drugs (NSAIDs)
- ✓ Sleeping pills and tranquilizers

How these drugs stimulate weight gain varies with their mechanism of action. For example, beta-blockers work by blocking the beta receptors of fat cells. These receptors normally help release fat from the cells. When the receptors are blocked, you gain weight. Prednisone, a corticosteroid, is five times more potent than the natural cortisol it's related to, with much the same action as the hormone.

Drugs also may cause weight gain indirectly. Side effects such as headaches, fatigue, and joint pain may keep you from exercising or preparing healthful meals.

If you are currently taking any medications—including birth control pills, ERT/HRT, and even drugs not listed above—*do not stop taking them;* if you suspect that they are causing weight gain, you must consult with your physician. Explore alternatives; many drugs are available in lower doses or in different forms (e.g., patch, pill, or injection), or a natural form may replace a synthetic product. Know and weigh the benefits of the medication versus weight gain and any other side effects you're experiencing.

And, of course, try the Fat Flush Plan. As I describe in the next section, various components of the plan are designed to target the weight you gain when fat's not fat. At the same time, with your hormones in balance, insulin under control, and key nutrients and oils included, you may find that you no longer need the medication you're taking. Acne may clear up without birth control pills; depression and fatigue caused by food sensitivities may improve, decreasing your need for antidepressants.

What the Fat Flush Plan Does When Fat Is Not Fat

The Fat Flush Plan targets water retention from the very first day. The cranberry juice and water beverage that you'll drink throughout the day in phase 1 is a powerful diuretic. Arbutin, an active ingredient of cranberries, pulls water out to be eliminated through your kidneys. At the same time, cranberry juice works on cellulite because, as we now know, the flavonoids in the fruit improve the strength and integrity of connective tissue and help keep your lymphatic system working smoothly.

Drinking 64 ounces of cran-water (in phase 1) and 48 ounces of plain water (in phases 2 and 3) will ensure that your kidneys and lymphatic system have the fluid they need to work properly to remove wastes and fat. Ideally, water should be filtered and noncarbonated. Water helps rid the body of waste, keeps tissues moist and lubricated, and may even help burn calories. The hot water with lemon juice you'll drink throughout the plan gives your kidneys another boost with lemon's diuretic action. And even the Fat Flush Plan exercise regimen, based on the minibouncer and brisk walking, has been designed to strengthen your lymphatic system and help rid your body of cellulite.

The plan's Long Life Cocktail, a blend of diluted cranberry juice and either psyllium or ground flaxseed taken twice a day swings a one-two punch of its own. Flaxseed is one of the richest sources of phytoestrogenic *lignans*. By binding to estrogen receptors and interfering with enzymes that convert various hormones to estrogen, flaxseed may help control estrogen dominance and the resulting water retention and weight gain.

In fact, many midlife women report that the flaxseed and GLA components of the plan act as natural hormone therapy, reducing hot flashes, mood swings, sleep disturbances, and tissue dryness without the side effects of fat-promoting synthetic estrogens and progestins. And for those Fat Flushers who are seeking even more individualized natural hormone therapy to replace their current drug prescriptions, there are health pharmacies all over the country which specialize in compounding tailormade natural hormone (see Chapter 12).

Daily portions of selected fruits and unlimited quantities of selected crunchy vegetables ensure that you'll get additional dietary fiber. According to B. A. Stoll, a high-fiber diet reduces recirculating estrogen by binding to excess estrogen and carrying it out of the body. You'll also find that the plan's various fiber sources will help you feel full.

By including 8 ounces or more of protein, up to two eggs, and high-protein whey powder, the plan prevents protein deficiency that can slow metabolism and cause cellulite and water retention. Without enough protein, your body loses muscle tissue, which slows metabolism. Pound for pound, muscle burns five times as many calories as other tissue. You'll find protein sources in the menus for all three daily meals because (1) your body needs the nutrient to rebuild tissue overnight, (2) protein helps you feel full, and (3) it helps avoid midday fatigue that can lead to overeating.

As you read through the recipes for phase 1, you'll notice that they do not include salt, but they do feature tasty herbs and spices. Sodium's water-retaining properties are well known, but you may be less familiar with the diuretic qualities of selected herbs. This is why the plan specifies parsley, cilantro, fennel, and anise.

Phase 1 eliminates two of the most reactive food groups, grains and dairy products. Following the two-week cleansing, phase 2 gradually reintroduces hypoallergenic carbohydrates. By keeping a journal (see Chapter 7), you'll be able to quickly identify any food reactions and make adjustments accordingly. In phase 3, your Lifestyle Eating Plan. Dairy and some grain-based foods are part of the menu, and you are encouraged to continue to note your body's responses, removing any reactive food permanently.

In phase 1, you'll not only avoid wheat and other grains, which can cause gluten intolerance and candidiasis, you'll also skip other *Candida* boosters—starches, sugars, and fermented flavor enhancers such as soy sauce. I have selected metabolism-boosting and diuretic herbs and spices such as dry mustard, cayenne, and garlic and mineral-rich apple cider vinegar to add flavor to my recipes without providing an environment for *Candida* to flourish.

HIDDEN FACTOR #3: FEAR OF EATING FAT

In Chapter 1 I explained how I came to learn about the benefits of gamma-linolenic acid (GLA) for good health and weight loss. You read about your need for essential fatty acids such as GLA. However, you still don't quite believe it, do you? Eating fat to get thin flies in the face of reason, of everything you've heard about the dangers of fat.

You're not alone in your fear of eating fat. An estimated 80 percent of Americans eat a diet deficient in essential fatty acids (EFAs). This is unfortunate, because our bodies cannot make EFAs. Yet, as precursors to hormone-like prostaglandins, they regulate *every* body function at the cellular level. This includes water retention, sodium balance, and fat metabolism.

In your efforts at weight control, fat also

✓ Carries fat-soluble vitamins A, D, E, and K through the bloodstream.
✓ Activates the flow of bile.
✓ Helps your body conserve protein.
✓ Slows the absorption of carbohydrates to balance blood sugar levels.
✓ Is a building block for production of estrogen, testosterone, and other hormones.

✓ Is a precursor for serotonin, which controls cravings and elevates your mood.

Every cell in your body is protected by a membrane that is composed largely of fat. Even your brain is 60 percent fat. Is it any wonder then that your body craves fat—any fat—when you eat a high-carbohydrate, low-fat diet?

Of course, the Fat Flush Plan does not suggest that you eat unlimited quantities of any fat. With the right fats, however, you'll end fat cravings, feel full, have more energy, and lose weight.

The Amazing Omegas

Two of the most important types of fat are the polyunsaturates omega-3 and omega-6. Alpha-linolenic acid (ALA) is the leading omega-3. It is found in cold-water fish, such as salmon, tuna, and cod, and their oils; in oils made from flaxseeds, hemp seeds, and walnuts; and in soybeans, wheat germ, sprouts, sea vegetables, and leafy greens. Omega-3 fats raise your metabolism, help flush water from your kidneys, and lower your triglyceride levels. These fatty acids also increase the activity of carnitine to help your body burn fat better. Studies in animals have shown that omega-3 fats even help prevent development of excessive numbers of fat cells when the fatty acids are consumed early in life.

Under ideal circumstances, your body converts the ALA into eicosapentaenoic acid (EPA), then into docosahexaenoic acid (DHA), and finally into prostaglandins. However, circumstances are seldom ideal. Excess sugar, a high intake of trans fats, stress, vitamin deficiencies, pollution, and viral infections are among the inhibitors of this transformation.

The omega-6 fat linoleic acid (LA) can be found in unheated unprocessed safflower, sunflower, and corn oil. Your body can convert the LA to GLA and arachidonic acid (AA) and then into prostaglandins, but as in the ALA conversion, many of the same saboteurs often interfere with this process. Thus, it is usually advisable to rely on the preformed GLA found in borage oil (24 percent GLA), evening primrose oil (8 to 10 percent GLA), or black currant seed oil (15 percent GLA). The omega-6 fatty acids stimulate your thyroid, thus raising your metabolism, and activate your brown adipose tissue (BAT) to burn fat rather than storing it in your white adipose tissue (WAT).

BAT is dense in mitochondria, giving the tissue its darker color. In mitochondria, nutrients are converted into a usable energy form through a set of reactions called *cellular respiration.* This stored energy form is called *adenosine triphosphate* (ATP). As I mentioned in Chapter 1, prostaglandins can augment the metabolic process called *ATPase,* which acts like a sodium-potassium pump to keep the right amounts of potassium in the cell and excess sodium out. The prostaglandin produced from GLA causes this sodium-potassium pump to burn even more calories.

BAT is high-energy fat. Its only job is to burn calories for heat. When properly activated, BAT can become your own fat-burning machine. The key words are *properly activated*. In thinner people, according to researchers, BAT is quite active. However, overweight people tend to have more sluggish brown fat. Age appears to be a factor as well, with BAT activity slowing down as we get older. Thermogenic vitamins, minerals, herbs, and amino acids can help stimulate brown fat activity.

About thirty prostaglandins are known, and they are categorized into three families. For each prostaglandin performing one function, there is another performing the opposite function. The prostaglandins produced from the omega-3 and omega-6 essential fatty acids perform different functions and must be kept in balance for good health and effective weight loss. GLA becomes PGE_1, an anti-inflammatory prostaglandin and diuretic. AA becomes PGE_2, which causes inflammation, triggers the kidneys to retain salt, and encourages water retention. PGE_3, produced from EPA, works with PGE_1 to control inflammation, along with blood clot prevention and other functions. All three are needed at various times; for example, if you cut yourself, you'll need the inflammatory action of PGE_2. However, to keep water retention under control, you need PGE_1 and PGE_3.

Omega-3 fats are burned off more quickly than other fatty acids, so when you diet, you lose omega-3s first—unless you include EFA supplements and food sources. This is just what the Fat Flush Plan does. Otherwise, if you lose weight at the expense of your omega-3 supplies, you'll find that you regain the weight easily and will have a hard time losing that regained weight. Your metabolism will have slowed because your body is less effective in using insulin when omega-3 fats are missing.

The New Kid on the Block

In the early 1980s, a research team headed by Michael Pariza, M.D. of the University of Wisconsin isolated a form of linoleic acid called *conjugated linoleic acid* (CLA). This fatty acid is produced by cows and other grazing farm animals from linoleic acid in the grass they eat. It comes into our food supply via meat, whole milk, and full-fat dairy products.

More than 300 studies, most in animals, have been reported since CLA's initial discovery, highlighting its promise in cardiac, cancer, and diabetes therapy. However, it is CLA's special properties for weight control that were the subject of the first human studies.

Dr. Pariza and Ola Gudmundsen, Ph.D. of the Scandinavian Clinical Research Facility in Kjeller, Norway, were among the researchers reporting at the American Chemical Society meeting in 2000. The American study of 80 overweight people found that those who took CLA when they dieted and regained the weight when the diet ended put the weight on as 50 percent muscle and 50 percent fat. Those who did not take CLA regained the weight as 75 percent fat and 25 percent muscle, the usual ratio of weight gain.

According to Dr. Pariza, whose team carried out the study, "CLA works by reducing the body's ability to store fat and promotes the use of stored fat for energy." CLA helps convert fat to lean muscle tissue, and muscle is one of your best metabolism enhancers.

The Norwegian study found that overweight people who did not diet but took CLA lost a small but significant amount of weight over a 12-week period. This study, also reported in the *Journal of Nutrition* in 2000, showed a stunning 20 percent decrease in body fat percentage, with an average loss of 7 pounds of fat in the group taking CLA without any diet changes.

Beyond the Fear

As I mentioned, your body converts EFAs from food into prostaglandins under ideal circumstances. However, circumstances often are far from ideal.

Our fear of fats, especially saturated fat, has driven us away from beef, dairy products, and butter. In their place, we've put refined vegetable oils, low-fat or no-fat dairy foods, and margarine. As a result, the balance of omega-3 and omega-6 fats is substantially skewed. We've also dangerously increased our consumption of trans fats, those damaged oil molecules produced when oils are heated or hydrogenated. Both results interfere with EFA conversion to prostaglandins. Other saboteurs include

- ✓ High sugar consumption
- ✓ Chronic alcohol consumption
- ✓ Smoking
- ✓ Use of cortisone or excessive antibiotic use
- ✓ Stress
- ✓ Pollution
- ✓ Vitamin deficiencies

Another change over the past twenty to thirty years has had a whole range of unforeseen (and perhaps some as yet unknown) consequences, including several affecting our intake of EFAs and CLA. Almost without our noticing, farmers and commercial food producers converted from feeding cattle grass to feeding them grains. Few of us would suspect this relatively simple and straightforward change to have the potential for long-term health consequences, but this now appears to be the case.

According to Jo Robinson, coauthor of *The Omega Diet* and author of *Why Grassfed Is Best!*, comparisons between the products of grass-fed and grain-fed cattle show just how much we've lost from our food supply:

- ✓ Meat from grass-fed animals has half the saturated fat of that from grain-fed animals.
- ✓ A 6-ounce steak from a grass-fed steer has almost 100 fewer calories than one from a grain-fed animal.

✓ Meat from grass-fed animals has two to six times more omega-3 fats than that from grain-fed animals.
✓ Cows grazing on grass pasture had 500 percent more CLA in their milk fat than cows fed the typical grain diet, according to a 1999 study reported in the *Journal of Dairy Science*.
✓ Chickens that feed on pasture have 21 percent less total fat, 30 percent less saturated fat, 28 percent fewer calories, and 100 percent more omega-3 fatty acids than do chickens given high-energy specialty feeds. The eggs of the pastured chickens have 400 percent more omega-3 fats.

The agricultural "advances" that have given us grain-fed cattle and chickens also have introduced synthetic hormones, antibiotics, pesticide residues, and additives into our food supply, having the potential to affect much more than our consumption and metabolism of fats.

What the Fat Flush Plan Does for Your Fear of Fat

Your selections for your daily proteins on the plan can provide some of the EFAs and CLA you need. I've even included suppliers of grass-fed beef in Chapter 12, Resources. However, I know that getting the proper balance of omega-3s, omega-6s, and CLA is so important to your successful weight loss that I've made specific oils and supplements integral to the plan.

Daily servings of flaxseed oil ensure that you get adequate supplies of the omega-3 ALA. Adding flaxseed oil to foods creates a feeling of fullness and satisfaction following a meal. The EFAs in the oil cause your stomach to retain food for a longer period of time compared with no-fat or low-fat foods. The physiologic effect is a slow, sustained rise in blood sugar and then a prolonged plateau. The net result is a corresponding feeling of stamina, energy, and satisfaction with no immediate hunger pangs to lure you into overeating.

Throughout the plan you'll take a daily supplement of GLA, made from evening primrose, borage, or black currant seed oil, and in phase 3 you'll add a CLA supplement. To ensure that your body makes the best use of these oils and supplements, the plan also eliminates or minimizes many of the saboteurs, including sugar, alcohol, vitamin deficiencies, and stress.

HIDDEN FACTOR #4: EXCESS INSULIN

After reading this far, you must be marveling at just how complex and interrelated your body systems are. Too much or too little of a key component disrupts the natural balance and you end up overweight, tired, and a victim of any of a wide range of diseases. Such is the case with the intricate system for metabolizing carbohydrates.

Putting Carbohydrates to Work

When you eat carbohydrates, glucose is released into your bloodstream. This signals the islets of Langerhans in the pancreas to produce insulin. This hormone takes some of the glucose to cells for immediate energy; it converts more glucose to a starchy version, glycogen. Glycogen is transported to the liver and muscle tissue for short-term storage, ready to be used quickly as blood sugar levels start to fall again. Short-term storage capacity is limited, however, so any remaining glucose is converted, again with the help of insulin, into triglycerides (body fat) for long-term storage.

When your blood sugar level drops, the islets produce the hormone glucagon. This hormone causes the glycogen stored in your liver to be released once again into your bloodstream and protein to be converted to glucose, all to restore your blood sugar level. Glucagon also releases fat from storage in your adipose tissue to be burned as fuel.

This process works very well when blood sugar is released slowly into the bloodstream, ensuring an equally controlled release of insulin. However, some carbohydrates are quickly converted to glucose, sending a flood into your bloodstream and triggering an equally high level of insulin. The excess insulin causes your blood sugar level to drop sharply, bringing on fatigue and cravings for more carbohydrates. When this happens repeatedly, a sequence of events is set off:

- ✓ Insulin levels remain high.
- ✓ Insulin struggles to convert all the glucose for storage but succeeds only partially; your weight increases.
- ✓ Cells no longer respond to insulin and refuse to store all the fat.
- ✓ Glucose that can't be converted to fat remains circulating in the bloodstream, wreaking havoc on your heart, kidneys, nerves, eyes, and blood vessels.

In the late 1980s, in a report in the journal *Diabetes*, Gerald Reaven, M.D., professor emeritus of medicine at Stanford University, gave this sequence a name, *insulin resistance.* Robert C. Atkins, M.D., author of *Dr. Atkins' Age-Defying Diet Revolution*, and others estimate that about 25 percent of apparently healthy, normal-weight individuals are affected by insulin resistance. If you're overweight, your chances are significantly higher. Possibly as many as 75 percent of overweight people are insulin resistant.

Not All Carbohydrates Are Created Equal

Carbohydrates—sugars, starch, and certain fibers—come primarily from plant foods, such as fruits, vegetables, grains, and beans. Milk products also contain some carbohydrates. Traditionally, nutritionists have categorized carbohydrates as either simple or complex based on their chemical structure. Sugars were simple and thought to be digested quickly to release high levels of glucose. Starches were complex and released glucose slowly as they were digested.

However, more recent research has increased our understanding about how food is metabolized, and the simple-complex categorization has been replaced with the *glycemic index*. This index lists foods based on the rate at which the carbohydrate breaks down as glucose into the bloodstream. High-glycemic foods are those that are rated 70 and up; moderate glycemic foods, from 40 to 69; and low-glycemic foods, 39 and below. Foods assigned a high glycemic index break down quickly and bring on a rapid insulin response. These include many refined carbohydrates such as white bread, bagels, rice cakes, and boxed cereals, as well as certain fruits and vegetables such as carrots, white potatoes, corn, apricots, and bananas. Lowest on the glycemic index are apples, cherries, grapefruit, plums, lentils, chickpeas, and yogurt.

Low-glycemic foods fill you up and help keep you satisfied longer. They also help you burn more body fat and less muscle tissue.

What the Fat Flush Plan Does for Excess Insulin

In a single generation we Americans have made significant changes in our diet. Among them, the percentage of fat in our average daily calorie intake has dropped from 36 to 34 percent. Unfortunately, this has been achieved largely by consuming low-fat, highly refined carbohydrates so obligingly created by food producers. To replace the fat, they filled their baked goods with sugar. We also eat much larger portions—megamuffins and megabagels, giant plates of pasta—again in the mistaken belief that low fat equals low calorie.

The Fat Flush Plan is designed to restore balance to your diet and to control your insulin levels. About 30 percent of your daily calories come from carbohydrates in the form of low-glycemic vegetables and fruits. Many are also high in vitamin C, which researchers at Arizona State University have shown delays the insulin response to glucose, and in fiber, which slows the release of glucose into the bloodstream. What you won't find, however, are sugar, bread, white potatoes, and other high-glycemic carbohydrates.

Low-glycemic foods such as those on the plan also have been shown to decrease your appetite, helping control caloric intake. In a study at Children's Hospital in Boston, overweight teenage boys ate 81 percent more calories on days when they ate high-glycemic instant oatmeal for two meals than on days when those meals consisted of a low-glycemic veggie omelet and fruit.

Another 30 percent of your calories come from protein. Protein stimulates the pancreas to produce glucagon, the hormone that counteracts insulin and mobilizes fat from storage. The beef and eggs are also valuable food sources of CLA, which has been shown in animal studies to improve glucose tolerance.

Finally, up to 40 percent of your calories come from high-quality fats, in particular, flaxseed oil. Its omega-3 fatty acids have been shown to reduce insulin resistance significantly in people with diabetes, according to a report by Australian researchers published in the *New England Journal of Medicine*. These researchers also found that the more saturated fatty acids (from hydrogenated oils and high-fat meats) found in a person's bloodstream, the more resistant that person is to insulin.

Studies have shown that consuming vinegar or lemon juice with meals can lower blood sugar by as much as 30 percent. The acidity in these foods helps slow stomach emptying, which means that food takes longer to reach your small intestine and bloodstream. Carbohydrates are digested more slowly, and glucose levels are thus lower. Thus the plan includes a daily drink of hot water and lemon juice and suggestions throughout the menus for using apple cider vinegar.

Speaking of flavorful additions to your meals, you'll find several herbs and spices regularly featured in the plan's recipes that boost your body's ability to metabolize sugar. Most prevalent is cinnamon. Researchers from the U.S. Department of Agriculture have shown that just ¼ to 1 teaspoonful of cinnamon with food metabolizes sugar up to twenty times better. Cloves, bay leaf, coriander, cayenne, dry mustard, and ginger lessen your risk of excess insulin by speeding your metabolism or by lowering glucose levels.

Among the plan's supplements you'll find not only the EFAs mentioned earlier but also several nutrients known to aid insulin action or regulate glucose. These include vitamins A, C, and E; magnesium; zinc; and chromium. Chromium is particularly important, yet our diets are frequently deficient in it. It acts as a transport mechanism to enable insulin to work more quickly and efficiently. Thus you store less fat and use more calories to build muscle. A 1998 study reported in *Current Therapeutic Research* found that individuals who took chromium supplements had an average weight loss of 6.2 pounds of body fat, whereas those taking a placebo lost 3.4 pounds. This weight loss represented a significant reduction in body fat for the chromium takers without their losing any lean body mass.

Once again, the plan's omission of saturated and trans fats, sugars, and refined carbohydrates will help its insulin-boosting components work at highest efficiency and effectiveness.

Even the exercise regimen, with the minitrampoline, brisk walking, and, in phase 3, weight training, helps keep your insulin levels low. You'll have fewer cravings for sugary foods, feel more energetic, be more alert, and lose the weight you want—and keep it off.

HIDDEN FACTOR #5: STRESS AS FAT MAKER

Living in this information age has most of us Americans going nonstop at "cyberspeed." So it's no surprise to me, after assessing my own clients' stress levels for so many years, that 68 percent of us admit to being stressed out—or that 90 percent of us admit to using food as our drug of choice to pacify things. The irony of the matter is that stress, as I suspected, is making the adrenals kick out certain hormones—such as cortisol, to be exact—that can cause you to gain weight.

Stress and Cortisol

In the early 1990s, noted researcher Pamela Peeke, M.D. spent three years at the National Institutes of Health examining the unsuspected side effect of stress: weight gain. Her work was published initially in 1995 in *The Annals of the New York Academy of Sciences.* Dr. Peeke discovered that stress makes you fat through a cycle of events that begins in the brain. The hypothalamus signals the nearby pituitary gland to release adrenocorticotropic hormone (ACTH). Then the adrenal gland, aware of ACTH in the blood, sends out stress hormones to handle things, including high levels of cortisol. Its job is to release glucose and fatty acids so that muscles have energy. However, after the stress moment has passed, the cortisol level remains high, stimulating your appetite to replenish fuel your body has burned. A high consumption of sugary foods prompts more cortisol production, causing the body to store more fat than needed, usually in the abdominal area. Dr. Peeke's work also indicates that if stress remains a problem, cortisol levels in the bloodstream will continue to rise, in which case the stress-fat cycle goes on indefinitely—along with those extra pounds.

In earlier eras, that enhanced appetite would have worked to your advantage. You would have burned through a substantial amount of calories running from a wild animal while hunting and gathering. Today, however, the type of stress you have to contend with is usually emotional—being stuck in traffic, juggling job and family, dealing with a difficult employer, computer crashes at critical moments, and so on. And as frustrating as all that is, it doesn't call for the same level of energy expenditure as earlier physical stresses, so now the calories you pile on are stored in your deep abdominal fat, ready for quick energy during the next crisis.

Psychology researcher Elissa S. Epel has confirmed and expanded on Dr. Peeke's findings, according to research published in the September-October 2000 edition of *Psycho-Somatic Medicine.* In Epel's research, fifty-nine premenopausal women, over several days, experienced a series of stress-filled tasks, from puzzles and math to public speaking. Interestingly, the women who felt the most stress were those with central fat, poundage behind the abdominal muscles. Not only did they demonstrate a tendency toward more stress, but they also produced more cortisol than the slimmer-tummied participants.

Cortisol activates enzymes to store fat when it contacts fat cells—any fat cells. Central fat cells are deep abdominal visceral cells, which are a fast energy source in times of stress. These central fat cells also happen to have four times more cortisol receptors than the fat cells found right beneath the skin. Consequently, cortisol is drawn to the central fat cells, which ultimately ups fat storage in that area. Thus, every time you're stressed, you're encouraging your body to have enough reserves of fat to handle the problem. This concept helps explain why chronic psychological stress, according to Epel, actually has an effect on body shape through fat distribution, creating what is commonly referred to as an "apple" body shape.

Apples and Pears

People with an apple body shape have a proportionally higher amount of fat around their abdomen than elsewhere on their body. On the other hand, a pear-shaped body carries its excess fat in the hips and thighs. Aesthetics aside, numerous studies have found that "apple" fat is associated with various serious illnesses, including heart disease, hypertension, and diabetes. Scientists believe that this association is again related to cortisol. The hormone causes fatty acids to be released into the bloodstream from the central fat cells. Because these cells are located close to the liver, these fatty acids race to the liver and put stress on the organ. Cholesterol, blood pressure, and insulin levels rise. The more central fat you have, the more often this fatty acid overload occurs. Before you know it, you are ill.

In examining apples versus pears and stress, Swedish endocrinologist Per Bjorntorp, M.D. suggests that the problem is in how we react to stress rather than the actual stress itself. He studied an entire town in Sweden, contacting those born in the first six months of 1944 or 1952. From the 80 percent who responded, Bjorntorp chose 284 men and 260 women, using their fat patterns as criteria. After the metabolic workup, the overweight individuals with intense cortisol responses had a substantial amount of apple fat. These same people were chronically stressed, having no motivation to overcome their problems. Captured in a type of extreme hormonal fatigue, they had stopped searching for any type of resolve to the reason for their stress. Bjorntorp likened this to posttraumatic stress syndrome. Similarly, women in Epel's study who demonstrated a defeatist response had elevated cortisol levels during stress and deeper apple fat. Many of these same individuals felt that their lives were spinning out of control.

Compounding Factors

Everyone handles stress differently. Some reach for a cigarette, some for a relaxing cocktail after work, and others for a hot cup of coffee. Interestingly, the more heavily a person smokes, the more visceral fat she or he has. About thirty minutes after a smoker puts out a cigarette, cortisol levels shoot up and remain high for at least another thirty minutes. In a study of 2000 smokers over age fifty years, the individuals who smoked the least were the thinnest. Alcohol has similar effects, raising cortisol levels and upping the amount of central fat. One Swedish study reported that nondrinkers had 38 percent visceral fat, whereas alcoholic men had 49 percent.

Caffeine isn't much better, since it actually helps extend cortisol secretion, besides promoting metabolic imbalances. Just 15 ounces of your favorite coffee contains enough caffeine to raise your epinephrine level by more than 200 percent. And that epinephrine pumps out more stress hormones, including cortisol. Chugging around three cups of coffee a day could cause your serum cortisol to stay at high levels eighteen out of every twenty-four hours, instead of just the couple of hours our bodies were designed to handle. Caffeine also promotes norepinephrine production. This stress hormone targets your nervous system and brain. Along with epinephrine, it increases your heart rate, raises your blood pressure, and stimulates your "fight or flight" stress response. In fact, caffeine actually reduces your threshold for stress so that you aren't able to handle it well. This might force you to cope by eating more comfort foods (invariably loaded with sugar and other high-glycemic carbohydrates), which creates more metabolic stress and fat storage. And remember, as I mentioned in the section on the liver toxicity factor, caffeine is in much more than coffee. It's found in over-the-counter medications (e.g., Anacin, Vivarin, and Vanquish), chocolate (e.g., baking chocolate, cocoa, and milk chocolate), sodas (e.g., Pepsi, Mountain Dew, Diet RC, and Tab), and tea.

Sleep and cortisol are entwined. Chronically high cortisol levels disturb moods and even sleep. Sleep deprivation has reached epidemic proportions in the United States. Today, almost 70 percent of all Americans report sleep-related problems—an astonishing 33 percent increase in just the last five years. And lab tests show that cortisol levels are much higher in sleep-deprived patients. A study published in 2000 by the University of Chicago's Department of Medicine revealed that not only does sleep deprivation affect tiredness and immunity, but too little sleep impairs the way your body handles food, creating impaired glucose tolerance. This can result in insulin resistance and obesity. It is believed that a lack of quality sleep, known as *deep* or *rapid-eye-movement sleep,* can impede surges of growth hormone, resulting in increased fat tissue and reduced muscle mass. Sleep deprivation, which causes lower body temperature and fatigue, usually leads to increased food consumption to boost energy and help you stay warm.

I've highlighted the effects of excess insulin on your weight. In his book *Sweet & Dangerous,* British researcher John Yudkin, M.D. examined another aspect of insulin, namely, its relationship with cortisol. He cited research that found that after two weeks of eating a high-sugar diet, volunteers had increased insulin and cortisol levels. Their fasting insulin levels rose 40 percent, but their cortisol levels shot up 300 to 400 percent! As we now know, cortisol works in concert with other chemicals to quicken fat storage and plump up cells, so controlling sugar consumption and getting a grip on insulin can help put a halt to excess fat.

There is another outside factor contributing to raised cortisol levels you should know about. Some prescription drugs contain cortisol more potent than what your body produces. One example is the corticosteroid prednisone, whose cortisol is five times more powerful than your body's.

What the Fat Flush Plan Does for Stress as Fat Maker

By now you'll recognize features of the Fat Flush Plan designed to control cortisol and stress fat, including

✓ Avoidance of caffeine, alcohol, and sugar, known cortisol boosters
✓ Protein at each meal to enhance fat burning
✓ Daily fat to reduce cravings and physiologic stress

As the preceding discussion makes plain, however, taking control of your weight involves more than taking control of your diet. The Fat Flush Plan incorporates various elements to manage stress, increase activity, and maintain cortisol at healthy levels.

The plan's moderate exercise regimen, based on the minitrampoline, brisk walking, and in phase 3, weight training to strengthen muscle mass, will help burn central fat and the fatty acids released during stress while increasing levels of the neurotransmitter hormone serotonin, which enhances mood and relaxation.

A full seven to eight hours of sleep each night is important to reduce fatigue, provide growth hormone to help burn fat, and reduce cortisol levels. I urge you to adopt a 10 P.M. "lights out" regimen to increase the likelihood of getting the sleep you need.

INSIDER TIP

I encourage you to listen to your favorite music during the day. Mitchell L. Gaynor, M.D. of the Cornell Center for Complementary and Integrative Medicine, has stated that you can lower your cortisol levels by as much as 25 percent when you listen to music for more than fifteen minutes a day.

Keeping a journal helps to identify the emotions behind your overeating. It also helps to release negative feelings and to provide a handy distraction when temptations arise. Many Fat Flushers have told me that by keeping a journal they are able to follow the plan even better and they now understand what triggers their overeating. Understanding the reasons behind your behavior is an important step in gaining self-control.

I encourage you to use many of the plan's features as the basis for rituals in your life. When exercise, journaling, and regular sleep are daily habits, they become integrated into your permanent lifestyle plan. During these activities, your mind's healing powers can help repair some of the day's stress damage. What a plan!

CHAPTER

3 The Fat Flush Plan: As Easy as 1–2–3

Among all the fine arts, one of the finest is that of painting the cheeks with health.

—JOHN RUSKIN

The Fat Flush Plan has a rather basic and clear-cut mission: to increase metabolism, flush out bloat, and speed up fat loss. At the core of the plan is the commitment to promote a balanced lifestyle and champion simple healthy habits that we all overlook or forget about as a result of life in our hectic twenty-first century. Every aspect of each phase of the plan is targeted like a guided missile to accomplish this goal: helpful essential fats [e.g., flaxseed oil, gamma-linolenic acid (GLA), and conjugated linoleic acid (CLA)], amounts of protein (8 ounces or more per day plus two eggs), antioxidant-rich vegetables, moderate amounts of fruits, calorie-burning herbs and spices (e.g., apple cider vinegar, mustard, cayenne, ginger, and cinnamon), cleansing diuretic beverages, exercise, journaling, and even sleep.

The Fat Flush Plan comprises real foods. It eliminates all weight loss–inhibiting foods and beverages such as white flour, white sugar, margarine, vegetable shortening, artificial sweeteners (e.g., aspartame), and caffeine in regular coffee, tea, chocolate, and many soft drinks.

In fact, the more meals you build around the Fat Flushing foods on the plan, the more weight you will lose and the healthier you will be. That's right. Hunger will stop, food cravings will disappear, and even depression will be a thing of the past, and triglyceride and cholesterol levels will balance out. Your circulation will increase, and you will look years younger as you feel reenergized, renewed, and refreshed.

The Fat Flush Plan is a springboard for a workable eating strategy. Each phase can be further individualized to target your personal needs by adding either more protein or more carbs sooner rather than later. For example, if you are a weight lifter or a large-framed, muscular individual, or if you have been suffering from severe stress due to an illness, you may need more than the 8 ounces of protein per day, perhaps even 12 ounces. Feel free to increase the meat, fish, poultry, or whey protein shake recommendations to fit your needs. Similarly, when you embark on the Two-Week Fat Flush but feel you absolutely must maintain your weekly two-hour or longer exercise schedule, then you may need to pop in a friendly carb or two right at the get-go.

The good news about the Fat Flush Plan is that you won't have to cut out your favorite foods forever or maintain a strict daily routine permanently. You just need to know the basic principles of Fat Flushing, which are discussed below, so that you can rely on the foods that will keep you lean with the help of the easy-to-follow menus and simple recipes.

My original Two-Week Fat Flush has been so wildly popular with clients and cyberspace visitors that I have fine-tuned and expanded the original program to maximize your results. You will have not only fourteen days of menus but more than twenty deliciously simple recipes to enjoy on the Two-Week Fat Flush. And you can always personalize any menu (breakfast, lunch, or dinner)—or recipe for that matter—to satisfy your own tastes based on the expanded lists of Fat Flushing foods provided.

I've also taken the program one step further to include an ongoing Fat Flush Program and a Lifestyle Eating Program. These are discussed below as phases 2 and 3.

Moreover, as so many of my clients have experienced, you can look forward to shedding unwanted pounds and feeling refreshed, cleansed, and nourished on all levels at every step of the plan. On the diet front, you will be putting a tight lid on and counteracting the effects of toxic foods, birth control pills, medications, and a stressful lifestyle. And this is important because your system likely has been overloaded and overburdened, creating havoc in your liver and lymph and decreasing your body's fat-burning ability. The Fat Flush Plan allows you to clean up and take control of your body and your life.

Here's what is in store for you to enjoy during every phase of the Fat Flush Plan:

✓ POWERFUL PROTEINS—with 8 ounces or more a day, such as eggs, lean beef, chicken, fish, and whey—boost metabolism by up to 25 percent for about twelve hours to keep metabolic fires burning. Proteins are the tissue and muscle rebuilders par excellence. For every pound of muscle gained, you burn an extra 70 calories per hour. Subsequently, you will help stop hunger and keep blood sugar/insulin levels steady as well as support your system's detoxification process. And you'll actually be eating eggs with yolks on the diet because the sulfur-bearing amino acids they contain help the liver metabolize fats.

✓ AMAZING OMEGAS—such as high-lignan flaxseed oil and GLA-rich botanicals from evening primrose oil, borage, or black currant seed oil—trigger fat burning rather than fat storage. Flaxseed oil tops the satiety scale and can attract oil-soluble poisons that have been lodged in your fat stores and transport them out of the system. The GLA oils can mobilize brown adipose tissue (BAT), which burns off excess calories and boosts energy.

✓ COLORFUL, FRIENDLY CARBOHYDRATES—such as antioxidant-rich fruits and veggies—that are high in natural enzymes, vitamins, and minerals such as potassium keep sodium out of your cells to banish water retention.

✓ THERMOGENIC SPICES—such as ginger, cayenne, mustard, and cinnamon—raise your body temperature and kick your metabolism into high gear. In fact, studies show that some of these seasonings triple the body's ability to burn calories for fuel rather than store them as fat.

✓ ELIMINATION OF METABOLISM BLOCKERS—such as wheat, milk, and yeast-based seasonings—to protect your fat-burning process and ward off those unsightly allergy-related symptoms, such as puffy eyes and dark circles under the eyes. Omitting them is vital to your weight loss success because they have a way of retaining fluid, slowing down metabolism, and making fat stick.

✓ LONG LIFE COCKTAIL—To increase elimination, you'll drink this refreshing mixture filled with emulsifying enzymes from unsweetened cranberry juice diluted with water to help digest those fatty globules in the lymphatic system—your body's fat disposal dump, discussed in detail in Chapter 2. The high-fiber additions of psyllium (or ground-up flaxseeds) to the cocktail block fat absorption, increase fat excretion, and bind toxins so that they are not reabsorbed into the body.

BEFORE YOU BEGIN

The week before you begin phase 1 is the best time to prepare your system for the Fat Flush Plan. Probably one of the most important preparations is to begin increasing your water intake between meals. Begin drinking at least two glasses between breakfast and lunch and two more between lunch and dinner. This will start increasing your hydration and create the new habit of power drinking to get more water into your system. After you feel confident that your hydration levels are increasing, begin to banish all trans fats from margarine, fried foods, and processed vegetable oils (see Chapter 4). Next, eliminate all the whites from your diet: white sugar, white rice, and white flour. Stock up instead on lots of fiber-rich veggies in all colors of the rainbow. Green, yellow, red, and orange veggies aid the cleansing process by providing natural fiber, which helps sweep out toxins, and pigment-based antioxidants that aid the liver by keeping its detox pathways on the move. Adding a couple of pieces of fresh fruit also will help cleansing because fruits are a rich source of enzyme-activating potassium that starts to move accumulated fluids from your tissues.

By far the most important thing you can do to prepare your system for the plan is to gradually taper off all alcohol, coffee, tea, colas, and soft drinks. This includes any regular or decaf or aspartame-sweetened beverages. As you learned in Chapter 2, even decaffeinated beverages have some caffeine, which stresses the liver and impedes its ability to break down fat. In addition, the acidity in decaffeinated coffee, for example, is higher than that in regular coffee because of the beans they use to make decaf. Add to this the rancid oils and chemicals such as trichlorothylene or methylene chloride (dry-cleaning chemicals) used in the decaffeinating process, and you can see why decaf coffee is not the Fat Flushing beverage of choice.

Thus, if you are a heavy coffee drinker (having more than two cups per day), here is what I suggest: Replace it with herbal coffees, which give you the taste and feel of the real McCoy. The herbal coffees I enjoy and serve to my heavy-duty coffee–drinking friends not only are flavorful and satisfying but also are brewed like real coffee. Although there may be more brands on the market, the one I typically use is called Teeccino (see Chapter 9).

I would cut down coffee consumption gradually by eliminating one cup every other day until you are down to just one cup a day, using the herbal coffees as a substitute for the other cups.

Taking these easy steps will help to prevent the withdrawal symptoms that about one in four Fat Flushers experience while on phase 1 during the first four days. Withdrawal from caffeine and sugar in particular can include such symptoms as headache, fatigue, irritability, and even increased hunger. These symptoms typically disappear by day five.

PHASE 1: THE TWO-WEEK FAT FLUSH

This kickoff phase, which is based on an average of 1100 to 1200 calories daily, is designed to jumpstart weight loss for dramatic results. This two-week phase will transform your shape by accelerating fat loss from your body's favorite fat storage areas—your hips, thighs, and buttocks. Some individuals report up to a loss of 12 inches during this first phase of the diet, whereas they may lose only 5 pounds. This means that they are losing fat and bloat, not muscle (as with so many other diet programs). Remember, muscle weighs more than fat, so dropping a couple of dress sizes can be more significant than losing 10 pounds on the scale.

Regardless of how much weight or how many inches you need to lose, everybody needs to start with phase 1. Why? Because we all need a good cleaning out in order to activate and support the fat-burning process. The Two-Week Fat Flush is a cleansing program first and foremost because cleansing helps to facilitate weight loss by giving your liver—the body's premier fat-burning organ—some well-deserved support and nourishment. By doing this, you'll help your liver's ability to break down fats more efficiently the way it was designed originally. Remember, as you learned in Chapter 2, a liver clogged with chemicals and poisons cannot perform its fat-burning duties. Many of my clients refer to this two-week phase rather affectionately as "Diet Boot Camp." And I agree. It is a program that is especially motivating if you have had difficulty losing weight before or if you have a lot of weight to lose. Period.

While fat can be burned off by eating the proper foods, taking thermogenic agents, and exercising, other weight loss regimens rarely rid your body of stored toxins. Unburned poisons often migrate from the shrinking fat reserves to the bloodstream, organs, and tissues, causing discomfort such as headache, irritability, and nausea. This is why most people find it difficult to stay on other weight loss programs and wind up not feeling well.

Phase 1, the Two-Week Fat Flush, counters this quite effectively by increasing oil (in the form of flaxseed oil), fiber, water, and exercise. While fiber, water, and exercise can flush out toxins through the bowels, urine, and sweat, the oil can attract oil-soluble toxins that have been lodged in the fatty tissues of the body and carry them out of the system for elimination too.

Now, if you have a lot of weight to lose (over 25 pounds), you can stay on the initial phase of the program longer than two weeks. In fact, up to one month would be safe—but a little boring, to tell you the truth, because your food choices would be so limited. You may have more success moving to phase 2, where your weight loss will slow somewhat but you will have a greater variety of foods from which to choose. Please note that phase 1 of this program is a bit too severe and rigorous for individuals who have kidney or liver disease, are pregnant or breastfeeding, have a history of eating disorders, or are under age twelve.

PHASE 2: THE ONGOING FAT FLUSH

Phase 2, the Ongoing Fat Flush, is the next step for those individuals who have additional weight to lose but who also want to pursue a more moderate cleansing program and enjoy a bit more variety in food choices while still losing weight. This phase 2 program is designed for ongoing weight loss, with 1200 to 1500 calories each day, and is designed to be followed until you reach your desired weight or size.

Phase 2 is the perfect transition for those who are moving toward but are not quite ready for a lifestyle eating regimen. The Ongoing Fat Flush includes the foundational Fat Flushing foods from phase 1 with the addition of up to two friendly carbohydrate choices put back into the menu plan one at a time each week. Easing them in this way will help you to determine whether the new food is helping or hindering your weight loss goals.

Interestingly, some individuals may notice a slowdown in weight loss because of the additional carbohydrates, whereas others progress at the same rate as in phase 1. I recommend that you stay on phase 2 until you have achieved or nearly achieved your weight goal. For some, this may mean two weeks; for others, it may mean another four to six weeks; and for still others with a lot of weight to lose, it may mean months.

Journaling at this transition time is absolutely key. If you start adding on a pound or two, you will be able to track this immediately and cut out or reduce the amount of the offending food before it becomes a real challenge. Journaling also will help you in the phase 3 lifestyle plan to track which foods you can't tolerate. Symptoms such as bloating, gas, drowsiness, and the return of cravings are your body's private distress signals that should spur you on to take action—immediately!

And keep in mind that you can always go back to phase 1 if you need the structure of a more disciplined regimen.

PHASE 3: THE LIFESTYLE EATING PLAN

Phase 3, the Lifestyle Eating Plan, is really the Fat Flush maintenance program for lifetime weight control. This phase offers over 1500 calories daily, providing a basic lifelong eating program designed to increase your vitality and well-being for life. At this time, you will be using phase 2 as your foundational program, with its one or two friendly carb choices. You can now add up to two dairy products as well as two more friendly carbs, making the grand total up to four friendly carbs—weight permitting. Phase 3 friendly carbs include more choices from a variety of starchier veggies and nongluten hypoallergenic grains. As in phase 2, you will add these latest foods one at a time to make sure that you are tolerating the new additions without any allergic symptoms.

Phase 3, I believe, is more appropriate for both pregnant and breastfeeding women because of the higher calorie and calcium content from the additional starchy and nongluten grains and dairy products. My experience on the Fat Flush Plan has taught me that although leafy greens are also rich in calcium—for example, ½ cup of collard greens or turnip greens contains about 250 milligrams (mg) of calcium, compared with a cup of milk at 300 mg of calcium—and are widely available in all phases of the program, most dieters prefer dairy calcium. And it makes menu planning a heck of a lot easier.

However, if you have noticed that cellulite has disappeared because you have avoided all dairy products on the other phases and are reluctant to put dairy back in your diet, I would suggest that you cover your calcium bases with a low-dose calcium supplement. Take twice as much magnesium to ensure absorption and utilization.

To make sure that you don't gain back fat even if you gain back some weight during the phase 3 lifestyle program, the supplement CLA will be introduced. Remember that clinical trial I told you about in Chapter 2? In a research study in which one of eighty overweight people who dieted had regained weight, it was discovered that those who took CLA put the pounds back on in a ratio of half fat to half muscle.

ALL THREE PHASES

To optimize the results of your diet and exercise program on all phases of the plan, powerful nutrients that cleanse, support, and regenerate the liver as well as those which enhance both fat and carbohydrate metabolism are also recommended. These include dandelion root, milk thistle, Oregon grape root, methionine, inositol, choline, lipase, chromium, and the nutrient L-carnitine, an amino acid shown to raise the body's fat-burning ability eleven times.

The Power of Ritual

Once you experience the cleansing aspect in the initial phases of the plan, you'll probably discover that you think more clearly and are more mentally alert. As one first-time Fat Flusher remarked, "We can't expect to have sharp minds and luminous spirits when our bodies are polluted." Many devotees find that when their bodies are cleansed, they are more willing—and better prepared—to deal with other facets of their being.

Because the Fat Flush Plan was designed originally as a seasonal tuneup, done four times a year at designated times, it taps into the power of ritual. Its practical, systemized approach not only creates a sense of order but also is reassuring when it is so easy to become confused and overwhelmed by the sheer choices of eating plans.

Tuning in to Your Deeper Side

You'll discover journaling to be a vital companion to your Fat Flush experience. It helps you keep tabs on your food and eating habits. As a matter of fact, this in itself has been shown to be enough to prevent weight gain according to some experts. Your Fat Flush journal helps you track your food consumption, food responses (e.g., bloating, drowsiness, irritability, and headaches), and progress.

This is why during all three phases I suggest that you record your measurements, since you may be losing inches faster than pounds. And this is good, because when you're losing inches, you are actually losing fat. And let's face it, fat loss—while still maintaining your lean body mass—rather than weight loss should be your main long-term goal. Once you graduate to phases 2 and 3, where you'll be adding friendly carbohydrates and some dairy, the journal will give you an opportunity to discover your body's distress signals, alerting you to negative food reactions.

However, I also believe that journaling nurtures your body and soul beyond the diet component. This is why you'll also be tracking emotions along the way, giving you a clear idea of the feelings behind your eating impulses so that you can handle them successfully. Journaling creates a safe, comfortable place where you can vent your feelings, chart your success, recognize patterns, and enter a private world of self-discovery. Because of this, journaling helps you eliminate one of the *five hidden weight gain factors* you've already read about in Chapter 2 that we all seem to share—stress! Besides, taking the time to write in your journal has been shown to actually reduce food consumption, which helps reduce your fat-gaining potential.

Tapping into the Power of Exercise

The exercise component of the Fat Flush Plan represents another progression beyond other exercise programs. The Fat Flush Exercise Plan (see Chapter 7), like the diet plan, centers around the lymphatic system, the body's built-in fat-processing plant. This secondary circulatory system is constructed of millions of tiny channels running through all parts of the body. The lymphatic channels transport all kinds of waste products and fats from the intestines to the blood and then to the cells, relying on muscle contractions for their flow via the thighs and arms. But the lymph doesn't have a pump like the heart, so it has to be "exercised" with either a bouncing action, deep breathing, or movement of the arms while walking briskly.

To help purify your lymph during all Fat Flush phases, you'll bounce on a minitrampoline or rebounder for five minutes a day to gently ease waste materials and fat out of the lymph. By cleansing the lymph through gentle pressure on the thighs, lymphatic drainage is activated and fatty cellulite deposits begin to disappear. The greatest thing about this lymph-moving exercise is that virtually anyone can do it regardless of age or physical challenges. For instance, individuals who can't walk can still benefit from this exercise by sitting on the rebounder while someone else bounces on it.

On all three levels of the Fat Flush Plan you'll enjoy moderate low-intensity exercise—starting with brisk walking done daily and later adding strength training twice a week to help tighten and tone the muscles. Strength training, in particular, will aid your weight loss efforts because it builds muscle (lean body mass), which is metabolically more active than fatty tissue. In phase 1 you'll do twenty minutes of brisk walking, dramatically swinging your arms back and forth to stimulate lymph flow and keep toxins moving. Then you'll graduate to thirty minutes in phase 2 and forty minutes in phase 3. Doing more than forty-five to sixty minutes every day is now considered too strenuous for the body, so on the Fat Flush Plan, less is definitely more for many reasons that you will discover.

Exercise keeps insulin levels low and can even improve your emotional health because it releases endorphins, those natural mood elevators in your brain that make you feel good. Without a doubt, you'll feel centered, focused, and more in control.

Learning the Beauty of Proper Slumber

You'll also discover the value of getting the proper amount of quality sleep. Sleep reduces cortisol production—a key ingredient to stress fat—and helps restore the body physically. Throughout the program, you'll have a set bedtime (that magical time of 10 P.M.) and wakeup time, leaving you refreshed eight hours later!

All these fundamental elements weave together a splendid tapestry reflecting all the beauty of a balanced lifestyle. And let's face it, that's something we twenty-first-century men and women definitely need.

All the slimming details of the Fat Flush Plan are discussed in the following chapters. So let's get started!

CHAPTER

4 Phase 1: The Two-Week Fat Flush

Food plays an important part in proper nutrition, but what you do to your foods and what your body does about them is the final answer.

—DR. HAZEL PARCELLS

The Two-Week Fat Flush is a quick-start weight loss plan that cleanses the accumulated fats in your tissues and liver and purges fluid buildup from your system. It also prevents new fats, in the form of triglycerides, from forming. This two-week program reestablishes a beneficial fat ratio for your body composition, which sets the stage for continuous fat burning and appetite control. The result is steady weight loss.

Without a doubt, weight loss is what pleases my Fat Flushers the most! In fact, one of my female participants, Jennifer K—who had over 30 pounds to lose after her pregnancy—reported an impressive loss of 15 pounds in just fourteen days. Now you might be saying to yourself that this was merely "water weight" destined to come back the way it does after every other diet. But this is not so with Fat Flush. You see, Jennifer remedied the underlying causes of her "water weight" during phase 1 (as explained in Chapter 2). Then she continued to lose weight in phase 2 because she was still avoiding the wheat products and sugary foods that packed on the pounds in the first place. Of course, some Fat Flushers lose as much as 12 inches while dropping just 5 pounds. This is actually a good sign, however, proving that fat cells are shrinking!

The key to your personal Fat Flush success is this: Right from the beginning, set a goal for yourself, and track your progress in your Fat Flush journal daily. I truly believe the adage that whatever your mind can conceive, you can achieve. So set different goals for each phase of the Fat Flush Plan. For instance, you can start with a goal related to whatever it is that is motivating you to change your eating habits. It may be to lose 3 inches around your hips, get rid of that cellulite in your thighs and buttocks, slim down your waistline or tummy, feel healthier and more energetic, get rid of bloating and water gain, cleanse your system, or any of the many other benefits that Fat Flush produces. Journaling will help you keep tabs along the way, mapping out an insightful, revealing chart that will encourage you.

Also please keep this in mind: If you are following the program mainly for weight loss, do yourself a favor and forget about hopping on the scale every day. Weigh yourself only once a week. People don't lose weight at the same rate, and you can get discouraged if you hit a plateau. Besides, on the Fat Flush Plan you will decrease your body fat as you proportionally increase your lean muscle tissue. Since muscle weighs more than fat, you will be able to completely redistribute your weight and sculpt a slimmer silhouette without a dramatic loss on the scale.

GIVING YOUR LIVER A VACATION

The Two-Week Fat Flush is very supportive to your liver—that terribly overworked, often overlooked fat-burning organ you read about in Chapter 2. This phase of the Fat Flush Plan provides complete nutritional support for all the liver's varied functions. Besides metabolizing fat (to slim you down) and lowering cholesterol, it's busy making and storing red blood cells, balancing hormones such as estrogen, bolstering your immunity, storing glycogen, and neutralizing all poisons. If poisons or excess fats clog your liver, it can't perform its fat-burning function.

TWO-WEEK FAT FLUSH PROGRAM

Only certain foods are allowed on this accelerated part of the plan. Use them for your breakfast, lunch, and dinner. As you will see, the list is made up of whole natural foods eaten without salt. Trans fats (in the form of margarine, processed vegetable oils, and shortening), caffeine, colas, diet sodas, alcohol, aspartame, and sugar are eliminated in addition to many spices, yeast-related vinegars (other than apple cider vinegar), soy sauce, prepared mustards, and barbecue sauces. These foods disrupt your liver by overloading the detoxification pathways, resulting in decreased fat burning. They also can stimulate fat-promoting insulin, which inhibits weight loss.

INSIDER TIP **The success of the Fat Flush Plan depends as much on what you don't eat as on what you do.**

The herbs and spices allowed in the menus are not there merely to enhance flavor. They are powerful diet aids that accelerate metabolism (e.g., cayenne, dried mustard, and ginger), assist digestion (e.g., dill, garlic, anise, and fennel), improve insulin and glucose levels (e.g., cinnamon, cloves, bay leaves, and coriander), remove water weight (e.g., parsley, cilantro, fennel, anise, and apple cider vinegar), and protect against disease (cumin).

I encourage you to avoid extremely hot spices such as curries and chili peppers (cayenne is not a chili), because these types of seasonings can trigger water retention. In addition, many people get sleepy after consuming them. Similarly, black pepper is omitted because of its effect on the cellular pH, causing fatigue and drowsiness.

For this first two-week period, you also should avoid oils and fats of any kind other than the daily flaxseed oil and essential fatty acid supplement from gamma-linolenic acid (GLA).

Use low-sodium or no-salt-added chicken, beef, and vegetables broths (see Chapter 9 for specific brands) for sautéing, basting, and making those eggs in the morning. They add surprising flavor to just about everything, especially those leafy greens you see everywhere on the menus.

Cut out all grains, bread, cereal, and starchy vegetables such as potatoes, corn, peas, carrots, parsnips, pumpkin, winter squash, and beans. The gluten-based grains from wheat, rye, oats, and barley can be allergenic, creating water retention or "fat that is not fat." Others—the ones I call "friendly carbohydrates," such as peas, winter squash, and beans—will be added back gradually in phases 2 and 3, along with an additional carrot allowance.

You also will notice that, for now at least, dairy products (with the exception of whey), such as milk, yogurt, and cheeses, are off limits. Dairy is one of the top five food allergens. The calcium in the Fat Flush Plan will be coming from the best nondairy sources—greens! The highest-calcium greens are kale, collards, escarole, watercress, broccoli, and mustard and turnip greens. I would recommend getting acquainted with at least two of these leafy vegetables and rotating them into your menus. They are great sources of purifying chlorophyll and the most important mineral I know of—magnesium—for beautiful bones, strong nerves, cleansing, and elimination, not to mention at least 350 biochemical processes.

In the first two weeks, I not only dropped fifteen pounds but I was able to wear one of my favorite outfits again. What really amazed me was how Fat Flush removed those cravings I used to wrestle with . . . I was a grazer and a craver! Everywhere I go, people tell me I look ten years younger. . . . Even my nails are stronger.

My profession is demanding, and I count on having the energy and stamina to stay on top. I own, produce, and do a radio show, which means a tremendous amount of work every day. Fat Flush revved up my energy levels and helped me keep in the game. If I can successfully work this remarkable program into my busy schedule—anyone can.

On my show, I've interviewed all the top diet gurus and tried their approaches—from Suzanne Somers to Dr. Atkins. I can honestly say that I've never had such dramatic results on any other program. It really jumpstarts weight loss.

—Frankie Boyer, Host of The Business of Being Healthy with Frankie Boyer

TWO-WEEK DAILY PROTOCOL DIET

OIL

DAILY INTAKE: 1 tablespoon twice daily of organic high-lignan flaxseed oil

PURPOSE: Essential for its high–omega-3 fat-fighting and insulin-regulating potential

> **FLUSH FLASH**
>
> **One clever Fat Flusher carries her daily flaxseed oil in one of two empty film cases—the other is for the cider vinegar. Another Fat Flusher suggests keeping one bottle of flaxseed oil at home and one at work.**

LEAN PROTEIN

DAILY INTAKE: Up to 8 ounces per day

CHOOSE FROM: All varieties of fish, seafood, lean beef, veal, lamb, skinless turkey or chicken, and whey. Use organic or grass-fed meat whenever possible. Choose lactose-free, high-protein whey powders with about 20 grams of protein per serving and negligible carbohydrates. Consume tofu and/or tempeh up to two times per week.

PURPOSE: Protein raises metabolism by 25 percent and activates the liver's detoxifying enzymes.

EGGS

DAILY INTAKE: Up to 2 per day

PURPOSE: The omega-3–enriched eggs are not only delicious but also are brimming with antioxidants (e.g., lutein and zeaxanthin) for the eyes and brain, cholesterol-protective phosphatidylcholine, and sulfur to support your liver's cleansing process.

VEGETABLES

DAILY INTAKE: Unlimited (unless otherwise noted), raw or steamed

CHOOSE FROM: Asparagus, green beans, broccoli, brussels sprouts, cabbage, cauliflower, Chinese cabbage, carrots (one), cucumbers, daikon, eggplant, spinach, escarole, collard greens, kale, mustard greens, romaine lettuce, arugula, radicchio, endive, parsley, onions, chives, green and red bell peppers, jícama, mushrooms, olives (3), radishes, mung bean sprouts, okra, alfalfa sprouts, tomatoes, watercress, red or green loose-leaf lettuce, zucchini, yellow squash, water chestnuts, bamboo shoots, and garlic.

PURPOSE: These fibrous and colorful phytonutrient-rich vegetables will help speed your liver's cleansing and provide valuable carotenoids.

FRUITS

DAILY INTAKE: 2 whole portions daily

CHOOSE FROM: 1 small apple, ½ grapefruit, 1 small orange, 2 medium plums, 6 large strawberries, 10 large cherries, 1 nectarine, 1 peach, and 1 cup berries (blueberries, blackberries, and raspberries).

PURPOSE: Nature's natural cleansers are high in enzymes and minerals (e.g., potassium) and low on the glycemic index.

CRANBERRY WATER

DAILY INTAKE: 8 glasses per day

PURPOSE: The cranberry juice–water mixture eliminates water retention, cleanses accumulated wastes from the lymphatic system, and also helps to clean up cellulite.

HOW TO: To prepare cranberry water, purchase Knudsen's, Trader Joe's, or Mountain Sun's Unsweetened Cranberry Juice. Then get two empty 32-ounce bottles. Fill each 32-ounce water bottle with 4 ounces of unsweetened cranberry juice and 28 ounces of water.

FLUSH FLASH

To make cranberry juice yourself, here's a simple recipe. Put a 12-ounce bag of cranberries into a large saucepan. Add about 4 cups of purified water, and boil until all the berries pop. Strain the juice, and if you like, you can add a touch of Stevia Plus to take the edge off the tartness (brave souls can take it straight). This recipe makes about 32 ounces of straight cranberry juice, enough for about four days.

FLUSH FLASH

Buy only unsweetened cranberry juice—not the no-sugar-added kind. Such brands could contain corn syrup or aspartame.

LONG LIFE COCKTAIL

DAILY INTAKE: Taken 2 times daily: on arising and before bed

PURPOSE: To increase elimination and balance hormones

HOW TO: In 8 ounces of the cranberry water, add either 1 full teaspoon of powdered psyllium husks or 1 tablespoon of ground flaxseeds.

FLUSH FLASH

Be sure to mix the psyllium quickly and drink it immediately to prevent clumping. Also, this goes down best with a straw.

FLUSH FLASH

If you are taking birth control pills or any other type of prescription medication, make sure you take them at least two hours before or after the Long Life Cocktail. The fiber component can interfere with the absorption of medications.

FAT FLUSHING HERBS AND SPICES

DAILY INTAKE: To taste

CHOOSE FROM: Cayenne, dried mustard, cinnamon, ginger, dill, garlic, anise, fennel, cloves, bay leaves, coriander, parsley, cilantro, apple cider vinegar, and cumin.

PURPOSE: Metabolism boosters

LEGAL CHEAT

1 cup of organic coffee in the morning

SWEETENERS

DAILY INTAKE: Stevia Plus

WHAT MAKES IT ALLOWABLE: Stevia Plus is the *only*—and I mean the only—sweetener I will allow on the program. It is used in our morning smoothies, and it is an optional ingredient in several of the recipes for the Fat Flush Plan. (And yes, some Fat Flushers even sneak it into the cranberry juice–water mixture.) Stevia Plus does not affect blood sugar or raise fat-promoting insulin levels. And it doesn't feed yeast. The product's inclusion of the nutrient fructooligosaccharide (FOS for short) supports the good bacteria in the gut, ultimately aiding with total cleansing and liver support.

BESIDES THE DAILY DIET

BEFORE BREAKFAST: Drink an 8-ounce cup of hot water with the juice of ½ lemon to assist your kidneys and liver.

BREAKFAST AND DINNER: Take supplements rich in fat-burning GLA in a total daily amount of 360 to 400 mg per day.

CHOOSE FROM: Straight GLA supplements containing 90 mg per capsule (taking 2 capsules 2 times daily) or an equivalent such as evening primrose oil in 500-mg capsules with 40 to 45 mg of GLA per capsule (taking

4 capsules 2 times daily), or you may select borage oil instead, in 1000-mg capsules with 200 mg of GLA (taking 1 capsule 2 times a day).

DAILY: You also can take

- ✓ A BALANCED MULTIVITAMIN AND MINERAL SUPPLEMENT for general nutrition insurance
- ✓ A WEIGHT-LOSS FORMULA containing liver-supporting herbs such as dandelion root and milk thistle
- ✓ CARBOHYDRATE CONTROLLERS such as chromium
- ✓ FAT BURNERS such as L-carnitine, methionine, choline, inositol, lipase, and lecithin

Uni Key Health Systems (see Chapter 12) has been distributing a Fat Flush Kit for my clients and readers for over eight years. I couldn't find Fat Flushing supplements in the health food stores with all the right dosages or the right ingredients, so I developed this kit. I especially wanted to make sure that questionable ingredients with potentially harmful effects would be omitted (such as ephedra, guaraná, and gota kola) in the weight loss or fat-burner supplement. Other appropriate supplements are also listed in Chapter 12.

TWO-WEEK FAT FLUSH MENU PLAN

Here is a helpful fourteen-day menu program to get you going on Fat Flush. Each metabolism-boosting menu incorporates the nutritional philosophy conveyed in the preceding chapters. Breakfast, lunch, and dinner feature the best Fat Flushing, fat-burning, and diuretic foods, beverages, and seasonings. The more you build around these foods, the easier it will be to pare off the pounds.

Keep in mind that these menus are not set in stone. I know that many of you are working guys and gals, just like me. Although it's best to follow the menu plans as precisely as possible, you can always find something that will work if you're at a restaurant. Simply mirror the Fat Flush concept. This could be as easy as ordering something like salmon, turkey, a hamburger (without the bun), fresh seafood (e.g., crab, shrimp, scallops), steak, roast beef slices, or that old reliable standby, chicken—and then adding a side of veggies. Or order a Caesar salad without the croutons and dressing, asking the chef to toss in some onions and parsley. Then have it topped with some broiled shrimp, salmon, turkey, or chicken. Don't forget to "lemonize" when you add your flaxseed oil. Delicious. I encourage you to "lemonize" your salad by simply squeezing a lemon (or lime) over it instead of a restaurant dressing if you haven't brought your own.

Also be sure to put your personal touch to the menus. You can alter them to suit your individual taste. Just remember to refer to Chapter 9 and then exchange one food for another from the same food grouping.

Substitutions

Let's say you're not keen on kale. Not a problem. In fact, it's a great opportunity to expand your horizons and try some of the other great chlorophyll-rich greens listed. In fact, many (like kale) will be your main source of calcium on Fat Flush. Thus, if plain old lettuce has been your standard thing, be daring and live it up. Try arugula with its peppery-mustard flavor and radish-leaf appearance; bok choy, that mild-flavored Asian green; radicchio, the Italian red-leafed green with a faint bitter taste and crisp leaves; watercress, with its slight bitter, pepper-like taste; mustard greens, the dark-leaf greens with a pungent mustard taste; or one of the many other deliciously slimming and slightly bitter greens such as Belgian endive, romaine, red or green loose-leaf lettuce, spinach, or escarole. Blend different ones together—your tastebuds just might be pleasantly surprised.

INSIDER TIP **Recipes for the dishes in the menu plan that are marked with asterisks can be found in Chapter 10.**

I did the Two-Week Fat Flush and lost nine pounds in ten days. It wasn't hard to follow; it just become its own regimen. My energy remained good. I kept working out throughout. The short length of time really helped me stick to it without going crazy. After I finished Phase 1 I wasn't a slave to cravings. I did it for more than just weight loss. Your program was a great way for me to feel revived and renewed.

My friends have been impressed—they wanted to try it! I did receive compliments, and, most important to me, I could fit back into clothes that I hadn't been able to wear for a long time.

Maintenance has been important. If I go back up a few pounds, I go right back to Phase 1 for a few days. I feel like it's given me a base to work from.

—Ruth Rothstein

WEEK 1

DAY 1

On arising	Long Life Cocktail
Before breakfast	8 ounces of hot water with lemon juice
Breakfast	Veggie scramble: 2 scrambled eggs with spinach, green peppers, scallions, and parsley, and one 8-ounce glass of cran-water
Midmorning snack	½ large grapefruit
20 minutes before lunch	One 8-ounce glass of cran-water
Lunch	4 ounces of salmon with lemon and garlic, warm asparagus, mixed-green salad with broccoli florets and cucumber, 1 tablespoon flaxseed oil, and one 8-ounce glass of cran-water
Midafternoon	Two 8-ounce glasses of cran-water
4 P.M. snack	1 apple
20 minutes before dinner	One 8-ounce glass of cran-water
Dinner	4 ounces Cider Turkey with Mushrooms*; Savory Spaghetti Squash*; and grated daikon, carrot, and onion salad with ½ tablespoon flaxseed oil
Midevening	Long Life Cocktail

DAY 2

On arising	Long Life Cocktail
Before breakfast	8 ounces of hot water with lemon juice
Breakfast	Raspberry Smoothie*
Midmorning snack	1 hard-boiled egg
20 minutes before lunch	One 8-ounce glass of cran-water

Lunch	Beef Stir Fry: 4 ounces lean beef with greens, bok choy, mushrooms, water chestnuts, and bean sprouts stir-sautéed in broth with ½ teaspoon ginger and a dash of cayenne; romaine salad with cucumbers and sliced radishes with ½ tablespoon flaxseed oil; and one 8-ounce glass of cran-water
Midafternoon	Two 8-ounce glasses of cran-water
4 P.M. snack	1 nectarine
20 minutes before dinner	One 8-ounce glass of cran-water
Dinner	4 ounces of Parsley and Dill Snapper Fillets* and medley of snap peas, yellow squash, and escarole with ½ tablespoon flaxseed oil
Midevening	Long Life Cocktail

DAY 3

On arising	Long Life Cocktail
Before breakfast	8 ounces of hot water with lemon juice
Breakfast	Asparagus-mushroom omelet: 2 eggs, asparagus and mushrooms with a dash of cayenne, and one 8-ounce glass of cran-water
Midmorning snack	½ large grapefruit
20 minutes before lunch	One 8-ounce glass of cran-water
Lunch	4 ounces of broiled chicken marinated in lime juice with cilantro, steamed Swiss chard, and okra with ½ tablespoon flaxseed oil; shredded red and green cabbage with ½ tablespoon flaxseed oil; and one 8-ounce glass of cran-water
Midafternoon	Two 8-ounce glasses of cran-water
4 P.M. snack	1 pear

20 minutes before dinner	One 8-ounce glass of cran-water
Dinner	4 ounces of broiled sole brushed with low-sodium broth, parsley, and garlic; Marinated Artichoke Salad*; and steamed watercress with lemon
Midevening	Long Life Cocktail

DAY 4

On arising	Long Life Cocktail
Before breakfast	8 ounces of hot water with lemon juice
Breakfast	Blueberry Smoothie*
Midmorning snack	Celery, jícama, and carrot sticks
20 minutes before lunch	One 8-ounce glass of cran-water
Lunch	4 ounces of broiled shrimp with garlic and ginger; steamed broccoli with ½ tablespoon flaxseed oil; tomato, parsley, and cucumber salad with apple cider vinegar; and one 8-ounce glass of cran-water
Midafternoon	Two 8-ounce glasses of cran-water
4 P.M. snack	10 large cherries
20 minutes before dinner	One 8-ounce glass of cran-water
Dinner	4 ounces of Southwestern Flank Steak*; roasted red, orange, and yellow peppers brushed with broth; and collard greens stir-sautéed in vegetable broth with ½ tablespoon flaxseed oil
Midevening	Long Life Cocktail

DAY 5

On arising	Long Life Cocktail
Before breakfast	8 ounces of hot water with lemon juice

Breakfast	2 eggs over easy and topped with ½ tablespoon Homemade Salsa* and one 8-ounce glass of cran-water
Midmorning snack	½ large grapefruit
20 minutes before lunch	One 8-ounce glass of cran-water
Lunch	4 ounces of scallops sautéed in broth with scallions, minced garlic, and fresh parsley; warm green beans; tricolor salad of arugula, endive, and radicchio with 1 tablespoon flaxseed oil, and one 8-ounce glass of cran-water
Midafternoon	Two 8-ounce glasses of cran-water
4 P.M. snack	1 peach
20 minutes before dinner	One 8-ounce glass of cran-water
Dinner	4 ounces of Yummy Meatloaf*; pan-tossed zucchini, kale, onions, and tomatoes; mixed baby green salad with grated daikon and 1 tablespoon flaxseed oil
Midevening	Long Life Cocktail

DAY 6

On arising	Long Life Cocktail
Before breakfast	8 ounces of hot water with lemon juice
Breakfast	Strawberry Smoothie*
Midmorning snack	1 hard-boiled egg
20 minutes before lunch	One 8-ounce glass of cran-water
Lunch	4 ounces of broiled hamburger with onions and green peppers, tossed salad with grated carrots and cucumbers and 1 tablespoon flaxseed oil, and one 8-ounce glass of cran-water

Midafternoon	Two 8-ounce glasses of cran-water
4 P.M. snack	2 plums
20 minutes before dinner	One 8-ounce glass of cran-water
Dinner	Eggplant Delight*; steamed medley of yellow squash, water chestnuts, and asparagus; and greens sautéed in broth with garlic
Midevening	Long Life Cocktail

DAY 7

On arising	Long Life Cocktail
Before breakfast	8 ounces of hot water with lemon juice
Breakfast	2 eggs scrambled with red and green peppers and onions and one 8-ounce glass of cran-water
Midmorning snack	1 nectarine
20 minutes before lunch	One 8-ounce glass of cran-water
Lunch	4 ounces of tuna fish, green beans, cucumbers, and tomatoes on a bed of greens with 1 tablespoon flaxseed oil; steamed cauliflower and brussels sprouts; and one 8-ounce glass of cran-water
Midafternoon	Two 8-ounce glasses of cran-water
4 P.M. snack	10 large cherries
20 minutes before dinner	One 8-ounce glass of cran-water
Dinner	4 ounces of broiled lamb chops marinated in lemon juice, dried mustard, and garlic; steamed artichoke; Zesty Coleslaw*; and 1 tablespoon flaxseed oil
Midevening	Long Life Cocktail

WEEK 2

DAY 1

On arising	Long Life Cocktail
Before breakfast	8 ounces of hot water with lemon juice
Breakfast	Blackberry Smoothie*
Midmorning snack	1 hard-boiled egg
20 minutes before lunch	One 8-ounce glass of cran-water
Lunch	4 ounces of grilled turkey burger with fennel; steamed medley of broccoli, carrot, and cauliflower with 1 tablespoon flaxseed oil, parsley, and lemon; and one 8-ounce glass of cran-water
Midafternoon	Two 8-ounce glasses of cran-water
4 P.M. snack	1 nectarine
20 minutes before dinner	One 8-ounce glass of cran-water
Dinner	4 ounces of Cold Fish Salad,* warm asparagus with 1 tablespoon apple cider vinegar
Midevening	Long Life Cocktail

DAY 2

On arising	Long Life Cocktail
Before breakfast	8 ounces of hot water with lemon juice
Breakfast	2 scrambled eggs with cilantro, tomatoes, and a dash of cumin, and one 8-ounce glass of cran-water
Midmorning snack	1 pear
20 minutes before lunch	One 8-ounce glass of cran-water
Lunch	4 ounces of broiled sirloin with onions;

	spinach salad with alfalfa sprouts and red peppers, 1 tablespoon flaxseed oil, and lemon juice; and one 8-ounce glass of cran-water
Midafternoon	Two 8-ounce glasses of cran-water
4 P.M. snack	10 large cherries
20 minutes before dinner	One 8-ounce glass of cran-water
Dinner	4 ounces of Shrimp Creole* and steamed kale and water chestnuts with 1 tablespoon flaxseed oil
Midevening	Long Life Cocktail

DAY 3

On arising	Long Life Cocktail
Before breakfast	8 ounces of hot water with lemon juice
Breakfast	Peach Smoothie*
Midmorning snack	1 hard-boiled egg
20 minutes before lunch	One 8-ounce glass of cran-water
Lunch	4 ounces of grilled tuna steak brushed with broth; chopped parsley, tomatoes, and scallions with 1 tablespoon Refreshing Salad Dressing*; and one 8-ounce glass of cran-water
Midafternoon	Two 8-ounce glasses of cran-water
4 P.M. snack	1 apple
20 minutes before dinner	One 8-ounce glass of cran-water
Dinner	4 ounces of Chicken and Cabbage Supreme,* sautéed collard greens, and 1 carrot in vegetable broth with garlic
Midevening	Long Life Cocktail

DAY 4

On arising	Long Life Cocktail
Before breakfast	8 ounces of hot water with lemon juice
Breakfast	2 eggs scrambled with mushrooms, celery, scallions, and a dash of cayenne, and one 8-ounce glass of cran-water
Midmorning snack	½ large grapefruit
20 minutes before lunch	One 8-ounce glass of cran-water
Lunch	4 ounces of grilled tempeh with a dash of coriander; fresh radish and watercress salad with mung bean sprouts, one carrot, and cucumber slices; 1 tablespoon flaxseed oil; and one 8-ounce glass of cran-water
Midafternoon	Two 8-ounce glasses of cran-water
4 P.M. snack	6 large strawberries
20 minutes before dinner	One 8-ounce glass of cran-water
Dinner	4 ounces of Gingered Shrimp and Snow Pea Soup* and steamed yellow squash with 1 tablespoon flaxseed oil and ½ teaspoon cinnamon
Midevening:	Long Life Cocktail

DAY 5

On arising	Long Life Cocktail
Before breakfast	8 ounces of hot water with lemon juice
Breakfast	Raspberry Smoothie*
Midmorning snack	1 hard-boiled egg and broccoli and cauliflower florets
20 minutes before lunch	One 8-ounce glass of cran-water

Lunch	4 ounces of browned ground beef with ½ cup diced onions over escarole with 2 tablespoons of Homemade Salsa* and one 8-ounce glass of cran-water
Midafternoon	Two 8-ounce glasses of cran-water
4 P.M. snack	1 peach
20 minutes before dinner	One 8-ounce glass of cran-water
Dinner	4 ounces of Cumin Sautéed Scallops,* Roasted Veggie Medley,* and steamed kale with 1 tablespoon flaxseed oil
Midevening	Long Life Cocktail

DAY 6

On arising	Long Life Cocktail
Before breakfast	8 ounces of hot water with lemon juice
Breakfast	Spinach-dill omelet— 2 eggs, spinach, and fresh dill—and one 8-ounce glass of cran-water
Midmorning snack	½ grapefruit
20 minutes before lunch	One 8-ounce glass of cran-water
Lunch	4 ounces of broiled buffalo burger or chicken cutlet with herbs; steamed broccoli, zucchini, and okra with 1 tablespoon flaxseed oil; and one 8-ounce glass of cran-water
Midafternoon	Two 8-ounce glasses of cran-water
4 P.M. snack	1 apple
20 minutes before dinner	One 8-ounce glass of cran-water
Dinner	4 ounces of grilled halibut brushed with broth, dill, garlic, and lemon; Egg Drop Soup*; braised greens in broth; and 1 tablespoon flaxseed oil
Midevening	Long Life Cocktail

DAY 7

On arising	Long Life Cocktail
Before breakfast	8 ounces of hot water with lemon juice
Breakfast	Strawberry Smoothie*
Midmorning snack	2 plums
20 minutes before lunch	One 8-ounce glass of cran-water
Lunch	Warm Turkey and Spinach Salad,* steamed green beans with ½ cup jícama, and one 8-ounce glass of cran-water
Midafternoon	Two 8-ounce glasses of cran-water
4 P.M. snack	1 hard-boiled egg with cucumber slices
20 minutes before dinner	One 8-ounce glass of cran-water
Dinner	4 ounces of grilled lamb chop with a pinch of cinnamon and a dash of dried mustard, sautéed kale in broth, baked summer squash with a touch of cloves, and 1 tablespoon flaxseed oil
Midevening	Long Life Cocktail

CHAPTER

5 Phase 2: Ongoing Fat Flush

Give us this day our daily bread—free of strontium, mercury, and lead.

—ANONYMOUS

Congratulations! You just completed the most challenging phase of the entire Fat Flush Plan. Now it's time to step up to the next phase of Fat Flush. You'll continue to lose weight and maintain your cleansing momentum but at a slower pace. To accomplish this, you will be making a couple of changes.

First, you will replace the cran-water with pure spring water or purified bottled water. Since water is the most natural and gentle cleansing agent, the six glasses you'll have in addition to the water in the Long Life Cocktail and hot water–lemon juice mixture will help your kidneys continue their filtering tasks. In this way, your liver can begin to metabolize its own waste products without having to do the work of the kidneys. As you know quite well by now, metabolizing stored fat into energy is the liver's most important function. More water is the ticket to accelerating your liver's metabolic removal of stored fats, resulting in healthy weight loss.

But don't worry, you'll still be drinking unsweetened cranberry juice from phase 1, which helps to target cellulite. This time you'll have it in a half-and-half ratio with water in the Long Life Cocktail. The Long Life Cocktail still will be taken twice a day (on awakening and before bed).

The next change you'll love. You'll be adding one or two "friendly carbohydrates" back into your diet. And this means that you can have toast—from real bread! There are two or three breads I recommend in the Master Shopping List (Chapter 9). The first is a wheat-free, yeast-free spelt bread, made from sprouted grains and legumes, called HealthSeed Spelt. Sprouts (from grains and legumes, such as organic lentils, millet, barley, and soy) do not have the same biochemical components as mature plants. Although there is spelt flour in this bread and spelt is related to wheat, it contains less gluten. Thus, most wheat-sensitive individuals can tolerate it quite well. While these sprouted breads are not carb-free, the fact that the allergenic component is neutralized probably accounts for the fact that most individuals can handle a slice without gaining an ounce. In fact, I bet you will really look forward to biting into its chewy consistency and nutty flavor. The bread has flax, pumpkin, and sunflower seeds—providing the crunch value Fat Flushers seem to crave the most on the program.

Another choice is Ezekiel 4:9 bread, which many of my readers have used happily for years. The creator of this bread, Rainier Bakery, based it on the Biblical verse Ezekiel 4:9—"Take also unto thee wheat and barley and beans and lentils and millet and spelt, and put them in one vessel, and make bread of it." The bakery uses only organic grains and legumes in the original sprouting process. This process increases vitamins A and B as well as the minerals iron, calcium, magnesium, and potassium. The long sprouting breaks down the carbohydrates and proteins, making the bread easy to digest and assimilate.

You have to decide when and how you are going to expand your new friendly carb choices. After working with literally thousands of Fat Flushers, I can say from practical experience that your best bet is to add back just one friendly carb (such as a slice of toast in the morning) one day at a time and then track your weight responses in your Fat Flush journal. That way you will be able to pinpoint whether the addition of this single slice of sprouted toast is creating any negative response, such as gas, bloating, sleepiness after eating, or headaches.

Then add another friendly carb in the second week, noting your responses. These carbohydrates are the ones most unlikely to precipitate insulin response or weight gain. And they are also considered to be moderate on the glycemic index, which rates foods based on their effect on blood sugar.

For that second week, you may gradually reintroduce one of the following friendly carbs into your Fat Flush diet. I suggest beginning with just ¼ cup, journaling your reactions. If you experience any of the negative responses mentioned earlier, or if your clothes are a bit tight, then cut out that particular food immediately. You can choose from a sweet potato, green peas, cooked carrots, butternut squash, or acorn squash.

> *I have been on the Fat Flush diet for about a month and a half. . . . I feel like a new person. I have more energy and no longer suffer from bloating or tiredness. My moods are much more stabilized. Hooray for getting rid of wheat—I think that was the biggest thing I got from the plan.*
>
> —LYNNE LANGMAID

THE ONGOING FAT FLUSH DAILY PROTOCOL

OIL

DAILY INTAKE: Flaxseed oil, 1 tablespoon twice daily

LEAN PROTEIN

DAILY INTAKE: Up to 8 ounces per day

CHOOSE FROM: All varieties of fish, seafood, lean beef, veal, lamb, skinless turkey or chicken, and whey. Organic or grass-fed meat is best. Lactose-free 100 percent whey protein powders provide 20 grams of protein per serving. Tofu and tempeh may be used twice per week.

PURPOSE: Protein raises metabolism by 25 percent and activates the liver's detoxifying enzymes.

EGGS

DAILY INTAKE: Up to 2 per day

PURPOSE: The omega-3–enriched eggs not only are delicious but also are brimming with antioxidants (e.g., lutein and zeaxanthin) for the eyes and brain, and cholesterol-protective phosphatidylcholine and sulfur that support your liver's cleansing process.

VEGETABLES

DAILY INTAKE: Unlimited (unless otherwise noted), raw or steamed

CHOOSE FROM: Asparagus, green beans, broccoli, brussels sprouts, cabbage, cauliflower, Chinese cabbage, carrots (one), cucumbers, daikon, eggplant, spinach, escarole, collard greens, kale, mustard greens, romaine lettuce, arugula, radicchio, endive, parsley, onions, chives, green and red bell peppers, jícama, mushrooms, okra, olives (3), radishes, mung bean sprouts, alfalfa sprouts, tomatoes, watercress, red or green loose-leaf lettuce, zucchini, yellow squash, water chestnuts, bamboo shoots, and garlic.

PURPOSE: These fibrous and colorful phytonutrient-rich vegetables will help speed your liver's cleansing and provide valuable carotenoids.

FRIENDLY CARBOHYDRATES

DAILY INTAKE: Start with small increments (even half a serving), and work your way up gradually to the following portions, especially with the starchy vegetables:

Week 1, Phase 2: One serving per day
Week 2, Phase 2: Two servings per day

CHOOSE FROM: 1 slice sprouted-grain toast, 1 small sweet potato, ½ cup green peas, ½ cup cooked carrots, and ½ cup butternut or acorn squash.

FRUITS

DAILY INTAKE: Two whole portions daily

CHOOSE FROM: 1 small apple, ½ grapefruit, 1 small orange, 2 medium plums, 6 large strawberries, 10 large cherries, 1 nectarine, and 1 cup of blueberries, blackberries, or raspberries.

PURPOSE: Nature's natural cleansers are high in enzymes and minerals (e.g., potassium) and low on the glycemic index.

WATER

DAILY INTAKE: Drink 6 glasses of plain water per day for a total of 48 ounces per day.

LONG LIFE COCKTAIL

DAILY INTAKE: Taken twice daily: on arising and before bed.

PURPOSE: To increase elimination and balance hormones.

HOW TO (NOTE NEW RECIPE FOR PHASE): Mix 1 teaspoon of powdered psyllium husks or 1 tablespoon of flaxseed meal into 4 ounces unsweetened cranberry juice, and dilute with another 4 ounces of water.

FAT FLUSHING HERBS AND SPICES

DAILY INTAKE: To taste

CHOOSE FROM: Cayenne, dried mustard, cinnamon, ginger, dill, garlic, anise, fennel, cloves, bay leaves, coriander, parsley, cilantro, apple cider vinegar, and cumin.

PURPOSE: Metabolism boosters

LEGAL CHEAT

1 cup of organic coffee at breakfast (see Chapter 9)

SWEETENERS

DAILY INTAKE: Stevia Plus

BESIDES THE DAILY DIET

BEFORE BREAKFAST: Drink one 8-ounce cup of hot water with the juice of ½ lemon.

BREAKFAST AND DINNER: Take supplements rich in fat-burning gamma-linolenic acid (GLA).

CHOOSE FROM: Straight GLA supplements containing 90 mg per capsule (taking 2 capsules twice daily) or evening primrose oil in 500-mg capsules with 45 mg GLA per capsule (taking 4 capsules twice daily).

CONTINUE WITH: A balanced multivitamin and mineral supplement for broad-spectrum general nutrition insurance plus a weight loss formula containing liver-supporting herbs such as dandelion root and milk thistle, craving controllers such as chromium, and a fat burner such as carnitine, methionine, choline, inositol, lipase, or lecithin.

As mentioned in Chapter 4, Uni Key Health Systems (see Chapter 12) distributes a Fat Flush Kit that can be used in phase 2 as well as in the Two-Week Fat Flush. Check out the comparable Fat Flushing supplements listed in Chapter 12.

Use phase 1 as your foundational program, building on it with the phase 2 food list (see Chapter 9, "The Master Fat Flush Shopping List"). Here are some simple examples of how to "upgrade" breakfast and lunch for the Ongoing Fat Flush. You also may want to use the dinner menu ideas from phase 1.

BASIC BREAKFAST IDEAS FOR PHASE 2

Basic Fruit Smoothie

Make this your basic Fat Flush breakfast staple. Have fun and alternate or even combine allowed fruit to equal one portion.

Use ½ tablespoon of the flaxseed oil instead of the 1 tablespoon the recipe calls for, using the remaining ½ tablespoon to drizzle on your sprouted-grain toast. Your breakfast would go something like this:

- **Blueberry Smoothie**
- **One slice sprouted whole-grain toast with ½ tablespoon flaxseed oil and a dash of cinnamon**

or

- **Scrambled Eggs with Vegetables**
- **One slice sprouted whole-grain toast with ½ tablespoon flaxseed oil**

INSIDER TIP | Remember to divide your remaining flaxseed oil requirement for lunch or dinner in half.

BASIC LUNCH IDEAS FOR PHASE 2

4 ounces of broiled salmon
Leafy green salad with cucumbers, tomatoes, and lemon juice
½ cup your choice of carrots, peas, sweet potato, or squash with a touch of ginger and ½ tablespoon flaxseed oil

Once you are sure you are not going backward but continuing forward with your steady weight loss, add back another ¼ cup of your colorful friendly carbohydrate per week.

CHAPTER

6 Phase 3: The Lifestyle Eating Plan

Digestion exists for health, and health exists for life.

—G. K. CHESTERTON

Way to go—you have graduated to the Lifestyle Eating Plan. And this means that you have overcome many of your former eating habits, have stabilized your weight, and can better cope with real-life challenges. Hopefully, your journaling experience has revealed some emotional eating patterns that you are now better equipped to handle. Isn't it interesting that the fattening foods—the breads, pastas, mashed potatoes, and sweets—are the very ones we tend to gravitate toward when we need comfort foods?

The basic Fat Flush principles you embraced during the initial phases of the plan are still at work here with many welcome additions. This also will be an important time to continue tracking your food choices in your journal. This will help nip in the bud cravings or weight gain from *any* new food and facilitate its elimination pronto.

While there are some more liberal choices in the oil and fruit categories in phase 3, the most significant add-ons include dairy products and even more "friendly carbs" to choose from. Carbs such as brown rice, beans, baked potato, and corn on the cob are added to those you started to include during phase 2. Of course, this doesn't give you license to make a meal of just rice and beans or a baked potato (as you probably know by now). Measured amounts of these new friendly carbs can accompany your proteins and friendly fats in special combinations.

For the first week of phase 3, I suggest adding only one dairy product and eating it everyday that week. Note your responses in your journal. If you experience symptoms that may be due to dairy intolerance such as bloat, weight gain, gas, or phlegm, or if you have to clear your throat a lot, then omit that dairy product immediately. If not, keep your cheese and eat it too until you are enjoying two dairy servings per day.

During the second week of phase 3, substitute a new friendly carb for one of the carbs you are presently eating. Again, observe your responses.

Weight permitting, ultimately you can include up to four servings per day from each of the friendly carb selections.

And this leads me to another important aspect of phase 3 lifestyle eating—food combinations. The Lifestyle Eating Plan incorporates the Fat Flushing food combination rules I first learned about from my mentor Hazel Parcells, long before books using food-combining principles became popular. I have developed these guidelines further, based on my own experience with thousands of clients.

Dr. Parcells' research at the Sierra State University revealed that when foods were eaten in very precise combinations, people did not gain weight regardless of calorie count. In addition, gas, bloating, diarrhea, and constipation were greatly relieved.

THE FAT FLUSHING FOOD COMBINATION RULES

- ✓ ONE PROTEIN AT A MEAL. This means no double-protein combos. Have each individual protein food, such as beef, fish, poultry, seafood, or tofu, by itself. No mixtures such as shrimp and scallops or steak and lobster together at one meal. Digestion is impaired, and toxicity results.
- ✓ EGGS ARE THE EXCEPTION TO THE PROTEIN RULE. They are considered neutral and can be added to the above-mentioned proteins. They go particularly well with dairy products (as in a quiche) and add to the protein value of bean dishes. Eggs can be combined with a sprouted-grain starch (such as an omelet with HealthSeed toast).
- ✓ BEANS ARE CONSIDERED A STARCH/PROTEIN AND COMBINE WELL WITH DAIRY PRODUCTS AND VEGGIES BUT NOT WITH MEAT, FISH, OR CHICKEN.
- ✓ PROTEINS SUCH AS FISH, FOWL, AND BEEF DO NOT COMBINE WELL WITH GLUTEN-RICH GRAIN STARCHES (E.G., WHEAT, RYE, OATS, AND BARLEY). An example of this is a burger on a bun. Proteins do combine well with other friendly carbs, such as a baked potato, a sweet potato, corn, or peas—provided a green leafy salad is included in the meal.
- ✓ VEGETABLES AND FRUIT SHOULD NOT BE EATEN TOGETHER.
- ✓ MILK AND MEAT (E.G., A GLASS OF MILK AND A STEAK) SHOULDN'T BE CONSUMED TOGETHER. Dairy fats, however, such as butter, cream, and sour cream are regarded as fats and do combine with other protein foods (e.g., beef stroganoff).
- ✓ FLAXSEED OIL, BECAUSE OF ITS UNIQUE METABOLIC MAKEUP, COMBINES WELL WITH DAIRY (E.G., COTTAGE OR RICOTTA CHEESE AND YOGURT), FRIENDLY CARBS, AND VEGETABLES.
- ✓ WATER SHOULD NOT BE TAKEN WITH MEALS BEFORE FOOD IS SWALLOWED. While water is necessary for many metabolic processes, including digestion, saliva activity is weakened when large amounts of water are used to wash down food. Extremely hot or cold water depresses gastric juices and acts as a shock to the system.

THE LIFESTYLE EATING PROTOCOL

OIL

DAILY INTAKE: 1 tablespoon twice daily plus olive oil sprays for cooking

CHOOSE FROM: At least 1 tablespoon high-lignan flaxseed oil and 1 tablespoon olive, sesame, or rice bran oil per day. Rice bran oil has the highest cooking temperature of all cooking oils because it contains 42.5 mg of antioxidants per tablespoon.

BONUS FOODS: Enjoy a handful of almonds, walnuts or macadamias; a couple of tablespoons of seeds (e.g., pumpkin, sunflower, or sesame); half of a small avocado; or a tablespoon of nut butter if you are still hungry. A pat of butter, a smear of cream cheese, a tablespoon of mayo, or a dollop of sour cream is also permissible in this category.

LEAN PROTEIN

DAILY INTAKE: Up to 8 ounces per day

CHOOSE FROM: All varieties of fish, seafood, lean beef, veal, lamb, skinless turkey or chicken, and whey. Use organic or grass-fed meat whenever possible. Choose lactose-free high-protein whey powders with about 20 grams of protein per serving and negligible carbs. Use tofu and/or tempeh up to twice per week.

PURPOSE: Protein raises metabolism by 25 percent and activates the liver's detoxifying enzymes.

EGGS

DAILY INTAKE: Up to 2 per day

PURPOSE: The omega-3–enriched eggs are not only delicious but also are brimming with antioxidants (e.g., lutein and zeaxanthin) for the eyes and brain, and cholesterol-protective phosphatidylcholine and sulfur to support your liver's cleansing process.

VEGETABLES

DAILY INTAKE: Unlimited (unless otherwise noted), raw or steamed

CHOOSE FROM: Asparagus, green beans, broccoli, brussels sprouts, cabbage, cauliflower, Chinese cabbage, carrots (one), cucumbers, daikon, eggplant, spinach, escarole, collard greens, kale, mustard greens, romaine lettuce, arugula, radicchio, endive, parsley, onions, chives, green and red bell peppers, jícama, mushrooms, okra, olives (6), radishes, mung bean sprouts, alfalfa sprouts, tomatoes, watercress, red or green loose-leaf lettuce, zucchini, yellow squash, water chestnuts, bamboo shoots, and garlic.

PURPOSE: These fibrous and colorful phytonutrient-rich veggies will help speed your liver's cleansing and provide valuable carotenoids.

FRUITS

DAILY INTAKE: 2 portions daily

CHOOSE FROM: 1 small apple, ½ grapefruit, 1 small orange, 2 medium plums, 1 cup berries (e.g., strawberries, blueberries, blackberries, or raspberries), 10 large cherries, 1 nectarine, 1 peach, 1 small kiwi, ½ banana, and ½ cup melon (e.g., cantaloupe, honeydew, or watermelon)

PURPOSE: Nature's natural cleansers are high in enzymes and minerals (e.g., potassium) and low on the glycemic index.

DAIRY

DAILY INTAKE: Up to 2 servings per day

CHOOSE FROM: 1 ounce of hard cheese, ½ cup of low-fat cottage or ricotta cheese, or 1 cup of plain nonfat or low-fat yogurt.

FRIENDLY CARBOHYDRATES

DAILY INTAKE: Work up to 4 servings per day or as many servings as you can tolerate

Week 1, Phase 3: Substitute a new friendly carb for one of those from phase 2, adding no new servings, to gauge body's response.

Week 2, Phase 3: Add one serving, making 3 servings total per day, noting the body's response.

Week 3, Phase 3: Add one serving, making 4 servings total per day, noting the body's response.

CHOOSE FROM: 1 slice of sprouted-grain bread, 1 corn tortilla or a handful of blue corn chips, ½ cup peas, ½ cup cooked carrots, 1 small sweet potato, ½ cup acorn or butternut squash, 1 small corn on the cob, 1 small baked potato or ½ cup red potatoes, ½ cup chickpeas, pinto beans, black beans, or kidney beans, ½ cup brown rice or whole grain pasta, a handful of crackers, 3 cups popcorn.

INSIDER TIP

If bloating, gas, or weight gain are noted, omit the new carb serving and revert to the diet of the previous week. After the symptoms have subsided, add back ¼ cup (or other incremental amount) of a different carbohydrate and monitor your response until you reach your tolerance level.

WATER

Drink six eight-ounce glasses of plain water per day for a total of 48 ounces.

BEVERAGES

Drink herbal teas with no caffeine, dandelion root tea, or red tea (rooibos tea).

LONG LIFE COCKTAIL

DAILY INTAKE: Once daily, taken either when you wake up or before bedtime.

HOW TO: Mix 1 teaspoon of powdered psyllium husks or 1 tablespoon of ground-up flaxseed in 4 ounces of unsweetened cranberry juice, and dilute with another 4 ounces of water.

PURPOSE: To increase elimination and balance hormones.

FAT FLUSHING HERBS AND SPICES

DAILY INTAKE: To taste

CHOOSE FROM: Cayenne, dried mustard, cinnamon, ginger, dill, garlic, anise, fennel, cloves, bay leaves, coriander, parsley, cilantro, apple cider vinegar, and cumin. You also may add other flavorful spices and herbs as you wish, but keep these as your main focus.

PURPOSE: Metabolism boosting

SWEETENER

Stevia Plus

LEGAL CHEAT

1 cup of organic coffee at breakfast (see Chapter 9)

SALT

DAILY INTAKE: Not more than 1 teaspoon, or 500 to 2000 mg, per day (1 teaspoon equals about 2000 mg of sodium). Cardia Salt, a reduced-sodium salt with essential minerals such as potassium and magnesium, is the recommended salt for phase 3 lifestyle eating. Compared with regular salt, the sodium content of Cardia Salt has been cut from 590 to 269 mg per ¼ teaspoon, making it 54 percent lower (see Chapter 9). Sea salt or Celtic salt is also allowable.

BESIDES THE DAILY DIET

BEFORE BREAKFAST: Drink one 8-ounce cup of hot water with the juice of ½ of a lemon.

BEFORE ALL MEALS: Take a 1000-mg conjugated linoleic acid (CLA) capsule three times per day to maintain your fat-loss progress. As you recall from Chapter 2, CLA not only reduces the body's ability to deposit fat but also promotes the use of stored fat for energy.

CONTINUE TO: As you have done in phases 1 and 2, for breakfast and dinner take supplements rich in fat-burning gamma-linolenic acid (GLA) for a total amount of 360 to 400 mg per day. Choose from straight GLA supplements containing 90 mg per capsule (taking 2 capsules twice daily) or an equivalent such as evening primrose oil in 500-mg capsules with 45 to 50 mg of GLA per capsule (taking 4 capsules twice daily). Alternatively, choose borage oil in 1000-mg capsules with 200 mg of GLA per capsule (taking 1 capsule twice a day).

CONTINUE TO: Take the balanced multivitamin and mineral supplement for broad-spectrum general insurance plus a weight loss formula that aids in blood sugar stabilization, fat metabolism, and liver support. Such a formula should contain chromium, L-carnitine, methionine, choline, inositol, lipase, lecithin, and herbs such as dandelion root and milk thistle.

> *I have lost 13 pounds since I started the Fat Flush Plan. This may not sound like a lot, but it makes a big difference in my figure. I only have 6 more pounds to reach my goal. I will not be overweight when I reach menopause.*
>
> —*Meg Fischgrund*

THE LIFESTYLE EATING PLAN

Here is a two-week menu program to show you how to add back into your life all the new foods you have earned. Although I suggest that you introduce one new food per week, for the sake of more varied and creative menu planning, these two-week sample menus incorporate two dairy selections and just two friendly carbs—even though ultimately you can add up to four friendly carbs per day, weight permitting. The majority of individuals I have worked with seem to tolerate these amounts of dairy and friendly carbs without gaining weight or going backward. The portions are given in full, but you can always cut them in half and work up to the full amount. Keep using those veggie, chicken, and beef broths from phases 1 and 2 for veggie dishes (especially good with kale, collards, and bok choy) and eggs when the menu doesn't specify cooking oil such as olive or sesame oil. You may even enjoy a cup of herbal tea such as peppermint, Red Zinger, or fennel (good for the digestion) with your meals as long as the required water has been consumed.

FLUSH FLASH

Recipes for the dishes with asterisks can be found in Chapter 10.

WEEK 1

DAY 1

On arising	Long Life Cocktail
Before breakfast	8 ounces of hot water with lemon juice
Breakfast	1 cup of mixed berries with ½ cup of low-fat cottage cheese, 1 slice sprouted grain bread, and 1 tablespoon flaxseed oil
Midmorning snack	Handful of almonds
Lunch	4 ounces of poached salmon with lemon and dill, steamed green beans, 1 small baked potato with 1 pat of butter, and sliced tomato, lettuce, and parsley salad with apple cider vinegar
Midafternoon snack	1 apple and 1 ounce of Swiss cheese
Dinner	4 ounces of lean ground beef burger with sliced red onion and parsley, steamed cauliflower with dash of cumin, and mixed-green salad with 1 tablespoon of olive oil and lemon juice dressing

DAY 2

On arising	Long Life Cocktail
Before breakfast	8 ounces of hot water with lemon juice
Breakfast	½ grapefruit, 2 eggs scrambled with veggies and 1 slice of cheddar cheese, and 1 slice sprouted-grain bread with 1 tablespoon of flaxseed oil and a dash of cinnamon
Midmorning snack	1 tablespoon peanut butter on celery
Lunch	Salad Niçoise with 4 ounces of tuna, olives, green beans, tomatoes, and ½ cup red potatoes on romaine lettuce with 1 tablespoon of olive oil and lemon juice
Midafternoon snack	2 plums and 1 ounce of string cheese
Dinner	Chicken and Cabbage Supreme,* sautéed kale and button mushrooms with garlic, and mixed baby green salad with cucumbers and apple cider vinegar

DAY 3

On arising	Long Life Cocktail
Before breakfast	8 ounces of hot water with lemon juice
Breakfast	1 small kiwi and 4 walnut halves chopped in ½ cup of ricotta cheese
Midmorning snack	1 hard-boiled egg
Lunch	4 ounces of sardines (or mackerel fillets) with chopped tomato, parsley, and scallions and 1 small corn on the cob drizzled with 1 tablespoon of flaxseed oil
Midafternoon snack	2 plums and 1 ounce mozzarella cheese
Dinner	4 ounces of Tomato-Herb Veal,* sautéed chard and turnip greens in rice bran oil with toasted pumpkin seeds and apple cider vinegar, and 1 small sweet potato

DAY 4

On arising	Long Life Cocktail
Before breakfast	8 ounces of hot water with lemon juice
Breakfast	Peach Smoothie* and 1 slice sprouted grain bread
Midmorning snack	1 orange and 1 ounce of Swiss cheese
Lunch	4 ounces of broiled sea bass with lemon and garlic, sliced cucumbers and tomatoes with dill, and a handful of blue corn chips
Midafternoon snack	1 hard-boiled egg* and 1 ounce of cheddar cheese
Dinner	Rose's Special Soup* and arugula, endive, and radicchio salad with vinaigrette of 1 tablespoon sesame oil, roasted shallots, oregano, and fresh lemon juice

DAY 5

On arising:	Long Life Cocktail

Before breakfast	8 ounces of hot water with lemon juice
Breakfast	1 small kiwi, 2 poached eggs topped with 1 tablespoon of Homemade Salsa,* 1 warm corn tortilla, and 1 tablespoon flaxseed oil
Midmorning snack	1 cup plain yogurt with ¼ teaspoon vanilla extract and 1 tablespoon of toasted sunflower seeds
Lunch	4 ounces of grilled chicken breast with garlic and oregano, steamed green beans with slivered almonds, 1 small baked potato with chives and 1 pat of butter, and small spinach salad with 1 tablespoon of olive oil and lemon dressing
Midafternoon snack	10 cherries and 1 ounce of cheddar cheese
Dinner	4 ounces of Shrimp Creole,* ½ cup brown rice, and broccoli sautéed in 1 tablespoon of rice bran oil and dash of cayenne

DAY 6

On arising	Long Life Cocktail
Before breakfast	8 ounces of hot water with lemon juice
Breakfast	½ grapefruit and Weekend Turkey and Egg Bake*
Midmorning snack of peanut butter	½ cup of cantaloupe cubes and 1 tablespoon
Lunch	Tofu and vegetable stir-fry: 4 ounces of tofu, water chestnuts, bok choy, and bamboo shoots sautéed in 1 tablespoon of sesame oil, and ½ cup brown rice
Midafternoon snack	Carrot and celery sticks and 1 cup of cottage cheese
Dinner	4 ounces of Grilled Lamb Chops with Cinnamon and Coriander*; ½ cup of steamed peas with 1 tablespoon flaxseed oil;

	and romaine lettuce, hearts of palm, and tomato salad with apple cider vinegar and toasted sesame seeds

DAY 7

On arising	Long Life Cocktail
Before breakfast	8 ounces of hot water with lemon juice
Breakfast	Vegetable juice cocktail and Vegetable Frittata*
Midmorning snack	1 baked apple with 1½ ounces of goat cheese
Lunch	4 ounces of shredded crab meat in a small avocado with the juice of ½ lime and a sweet onion and celery salad with vinagrette of 1 tablespoon sesame oil, apple cider vinegar, and ginger
Midafternoon snack	Fruity Fruit Sorbet*
Dinner	Friendly Italian Wedding Soup,* vegetable melange of asparagus tips, ½ cup baby carrots, green beans drizzled with 1 tablespoon flaxseed oil

I had put on about 30 pounds, bringing my weight to somewhere between 190 and 192. Folks were gracious, saying things like, "You don't look fat." But I know how I felt and looked: sluggish, tired, old, and depressed. I never had a serious weight problem before 1996 and wasn't about to get used to it.

I have been on your plan for about thirteen weeks. The added bonus was the information about the GLA supplements, evening primrose oil, and lipotropic factors. I had always taken various vitamin and nutritional supplements and psyllium powder, but now I know what they do and why I am taking them.

I can't tell you how pleased and proud I am of my progress, I am down to 157 pounds. I have insurmountable energy, flexibility, mobility, and stamina. My tone and strength amaze me. I don't have to stop and rest when I am walking or carrying heavy items. Today I can wear my favorite clothes and have gotten rid of the big clothes. I'm looking forward to new-wardrobe shopping. But my ultimate joy is the fact that I can wear my favorite black dress again!

—Pam Jones

WEEK 2

DAY 1

Upon arising	Long Life Cocktail
Before breakfast	8 ounces of hot water with lemon juice
Breakfast	Banana Smoothie*
Midmorning snack	1 orange and 1 ounce cheddar cheese
Lunch	4 ounces tuna with lemon, cumin, and curry powder; 1 chopped hard boiled egg; steamed broccoli; and lettuce and tomato salad with apple cider vinegar
Midafternoon snack	½ cup chick peas and 1 ounce of Swiss cheese
Dinner	4 ounces broiled lamb patty with parsley and mint; ½ cup steamed peas, zucchini, and cabbage; leafy green salad with 1 tablespoon olive oil and lemon juice dressing

DAY 2

Upon arising	Long Life Cocktail
Before breakfast	8 ounces of hot water with lemon juice
Breakfast	1 cup strawberries with ½ cup of ricotta cheese, 1 slice sprouted grain toast with 1 tablespoon flaxseed oil and a touch of cinnamon
Midmorning snack	1 tablespoon almond butter on celery
Lunch	Rose's Special Soup* and spinach and red pepper salad with apple cider vinegar
Midafternoon snack	1 kiwi and 1 ounce mozzarella cheese
Dinner	Veggie tofu stir-fry: 4 ounces tofu, pea pods, 1 small sweet potato, red peppers, and water chestnuts sautéed in 1 tablespoon sesame oil; spaghetti squash with toasted sunflower seeds; and baby greens with lemon juice

DAY 3

Upon arising	Long Life Cocktail
Before breakfast	8 ounces of hot water with lemon juice
Breakfast	½ grapefruit, 2 hard-boiled eggs, and 1 corn tortilla with 1 tablespoon flaxseed oil
Midmorning snack	1 cup blueberries with 1 cup yogurt
Lunch	4 ounces salmon with dill and chopped parsley, onions, and tomatoes with lemon juice
Midafternoon snack	½ cup kidney beans and 1 ounce Swiss cheese
Dinner	Chicken and Cabbage Supreme*; collard greens, mushrooms, and olives sautéed in 1 tablespoon rice bran oil; and ½ cup brown rice

DAY 4

Upon arising	Long Life Cocktail
Before breakfast	8 ounces of hot water with lemon juice
Breakfast	1 cup mixed berries and 4 chopped walnut halves with ½ cup of cottage cheese and 1 tablespoon flaxseed oil
Midmorning snack	1 hard-boiled egg and 1 ounce Swiss cheese
Lunch	4 ounces lean hamburger with mushrooms, onions, and a touch of dried mustard; ½ cup cooked carrots with cinnamon; and sliced cucumbers and tomatoes with apple cider vinegar
Midafternoon snack	2 plums and 1 ounce string cheese
Dinner	4 ounces Shrimp Creole,* ½ cup acorn squash with 1 pat butter , and kale and tomato sautéed in 1 tablespoon olive oil with lemon and garlic

DAY 5

Upon arising	Long Life Cocktail
Before breakfast	8 ounces of hot water with lemon juice
Breakfast	Two (4 halves) Fat Flush "Deviled" Eggs,* 1 slice sprouted grain toast with ½ tablespoon flaxseed oil, and 1 tablespoon Homemade Salsa*
Midmorning snack	1 nectarine and 1 ounce goat cheese
Lunch	4 ounces grilled tempeh with cumin, garlic, and onions; baked cauliflower and toasted pumpkin seeds; and romaine lettuce with cider vinegar dressing
Midafternoon snack	10 cherries and 1 ounce mozzarella
Dinner	4 ounces baked halibut with lemon, parsley, and ginger; 1 baked potato with a dollop of sour cream, and spinach sautéed in 1 tablespoon olive oil with garlic and onions and a dash of cayenne

DAY 6

Upon arising	Long Life Cocktail
Before breakfast	8 ounces of hot water with lemon juice
Breakfast	Vegetable juice cocktail and Vegetable Frittata*
Midmorning snack	1 peach and ½ ounce cheddar cheese
Lunch	4 ounces of chicken salad with tarragon and 1 tablespoon mayo, steamed artichoke and ½ cup peas with 1 tablespoon flaxseed oil, and baby greens with lemon juice
Midafternoon snack	½ banana with ½ cup cottage cheese
Dinner	Steak and veggie stir-fry: 4 ounces flank steak, bean sprouts, bamboo shoots, red peppers, and garlic sautéed in 1 tablespoon

	sesame oil; 1 small corn on the cob; and a leafy green salad

DAY 7

Upon arising	Long Life Cocktail
Before breakfast	Hot water with lemon juice
Breakfast	Vegetable juice cocktail and Weekend Turkey and Egg Bake*
Midmorning snack	½ cup of melon cubes and ½ cup ricotta cheese
Lunch	Friendly Italian Wedding Soup*; ½ cup brown rice; sweet onion and celery salad with 1 tablespoon sesame oil, apple cider vinegar, and ginger
Midafternoon snack	1 apple and 1 ounce mozzarella
Dinner	4 ounces of broiled sea bass with lemon, ginger, and cayenne; warm asparagus; 1 small sweet potato drizzled with 1 tablespoon flaxseed oil

> *I have lost about 20 pounds in about two months on the Fat Flush Plan. When I had consulted my doctor about losing weight, he told me in not so many words, "Forget about it, women your age cannot lose weight." (I am fifty-eight years old.) This diet proved him wrong!*
>
> —CAROLINE KAMIYAMA

CHAPTER

7 The Power of Ritual

Reconciliation takes place within ourselves.

—THICH NHAT HANH

Now that you understand the foundation of the Fat Flush Plan, let me introduce you to another level of the program. Three distinct rituals—moderate exercise, sleep, and journaling—are included to help maximize your individual weight loss journey. Practicing them faithfully will empower you to do your best and reach your goals—and feel and look better than ever!

These Fat Flush rituals also will help you accomplish something equally important: the basic nurturing of your body. This means giving yourself permission to enjoy the full gamut of self-care, from health-promoting food and physical fitness to stress relief and proper sleep.

Reclaiming the right to care for yourself is fundamental to a successful, rewarding life. It also is the stepping stone toward enjoying positive, meaningful interactions with others. Nurturing your Fat Flush experience with these prime rituals will help you to stay focused, reduce stress, and develop better lifestyle management habits so that you don't have to be on a perpetual diet for the rest of your life. And isn't that a welcomed relief?

EXERCISE

When it comes to exercising on the Fat Flush Plan, less is definitely more—and with good reason. Regular, moderate exercise heightens endurance, increases muscle tone and flexibility, and encourages disease resistance. Bumping up your workout to a more strenuous level, however, doesn't increase these benefits. In fact, mounting evidence suggests that strenuous exercise can endanger your health—it can even be deadly.

This is especially true for women. Getting more than two hours of strenuous, nonstop activity on a daily basis can impede estrogen production (like menopause) and result in a loss of calcium, particularly in thin or slight-framed women. And even if exercise is reduced and estrogen levels become more regulated, a woman is still left with a 20 percent bone loss. Repeating this cycle along with a diet rich in mineral "robbers" (such as sugar, coffee, and soda) creates a stage for premature bone thinning before menopause even starts. This is one of the reasons why moderation is the key to smart exercise and diet during your twenties and thirties—before you cross the threshold of the forties and fifties, where the bone-protecting benefits of estrogen and progesterone wane.

There are, however, other reasons why overexercising isn't such a good idea for women. Maintaining a strenuous workout regimen increases the loss of body fat, which forces hormones to plummet. If a hormonal deficiency occurs, bone loss can be expected. Also, the increase in fat loss drains estrogen stores, producing irregular menses or a cessation of menses altogether. You frequently will see this unfortunate scenario in professional athletes, such as body builders, runners, and ballet dancers, who are able to turn their periods on or off with a 3- to 5-pound weight gain or loss.

As a matter of fact, it would be wise for any woman who was active in athletics in her teens and twenties and who missed around one-third or more of her regular menses to have her bone density checked. It's not unusual for older women to confuse this hormonal imbalance resulting from overexercise with menopause.

Another factor in support of moderate workouts is that exercising augments oxidative stress in your body. This, in turn, creates free radicals—those unbalanced molecules that damage tissue in your body. High-intensity training generates a superabundance of these malevolent free radicals, found to be the cause of over fifty diseases. In time, they debilitate your immune system and make you more vulnerable to premature aging, heart attacks, cataracts, infections, and a number of cancers.

Startling research by Kenneth Cooper, M.D.—the "father" of the fitness movement and previous proponent of strenuous exercise—appears to strongly support these facts. President and founder of the Cooper Aerobics Center in Dallas, Texas, he discovered that the damage done by free radicals generated during periods of overexercise could contribute to premature aging. His extensive findings were so revealing that he took a U-turn from his earlier belief in hard workouts, declaring that only thirty minutes of low-intensity exercise three to four times per week actually is healthier. Cooper's research shows that low- to moderate-intensity exercise is just as beneficial as high-intensity exercise—but without the rigorous wear and tear on the system.

Cooper's groundbreaking work in his book, *The Antioxidant Revolution*, describes his concern over the early onset of cancer and untimely deaths of world-class and other highly trained athletes. Jim Fixx, the highly regarded marathon runner, is one such example. Fixx suddenly dropped dead after a 4-mile run in Vermont. According to his autopsy, his arteries were almost blocked. This probably sounds surprising for a man who ran 37,000 miles in nearly twenty years and 60 miles per week up until his death. The cause of his death could be traced back to an overproduction of exercise-induced free radicals, which can instigate coronary artery disease along with other deadly conditions.

One other reason you won't be doing strenuous exercises on the Fat Flush Plan is that your body will be undergoing cleansing as it sheds those extra pounds. It is important to conserve antioxidants rather than expel them through strenuous exercise because they are your best tool for helping cleanse your liver. Thus they are, in reality, your fat-burning friends. And since your caloric intake is lower on the first two phases of the program, you won't have the energy you need to tackle harder workouts. Instead, you will start with low to moderate activity designed to help you accelerate weight loss, and then you will graduate to a longer—yet moderately balanced—routine that includes weight resistance.

Fat Flush Exercise Plan

You'll find these exercises simple, enjoyable, effective, and healthy—the direct opposite of overexercising. And you can do them right at home, easily fitting them into your schedule. You'll start off with bouncing and brisk walking in phases 1 and 2 and then add weight training in phase 3. Here are some of the ways the Fat Flush Exercise Plan benefits your weight-loss goals:

- ✓ IT KEEPS CELLULAR WASTES MOVING, CAUSING BETTER ELIMINATION. In particular, the exercises targeting your lymph system help stop toxins from overrunning your body. You enjoy a sense of well-being and aren't prone to weight gain. Consequently, your liver can operate optimally doing what it does best: burn fat. Exercise also helps blood, nutrients, and fresh oxygen reach each body cell to keep your body humming along. It also aids digestion, absorption, metabolism, and food assimilation and improves enzyme stores.
- ✓ IT BURNS THROUGH CALORIES. A thirty-minute brisk walk burns 300 calories, adding up to 2100 calories a week. This is a sufficient amount to oxidize almost a pound of fat—or 35 pounds annually. And since exercise increases muscle mass, it further helps burn calories because muscle tissue uses more of them for energy.
- ✓ IT REVS UP YOUR METABOLISM, MAKING YOU FEEL REVITALIZED. Recent research indicates that aerobic routines keep your metabolism elevated for four to twelve hours after you quit exercising, burning nearly as many calories as your workout did. And when you exercise, your body releases natural mood elevators called endorphins. They make you feel good and in control, which reduces your potential for overeating because of depressed emotions.
- ✓ IT HELPS CURB CRAVINGS. According to a California State University study, going for a ten-minute brisk walk prior to every meal can quench those snack impulses. Exercising also suppresses those cravings tied to

depression and stress. It encourages serotonin, dopamine, and norepinephrine production; these neurotransmitters help tranquilize the body up to four hours after working out. Anxiety is relieved, and you keep your appetite in control. In addition, exercise reduces blood sugar levels, increasing the effectiveness of insulin for muscle and fat cells. Steady blood sugar levels reduce the desire to snack on those problem carbohydrates and prevent insulin-related fat storage.

✓ **IT BUMPS UP YOUR ENERGY LEVEL.** It enhances your circulation and stimulates hormone production, such as testosterone, which invigorates everyone—men and women. When your body is energized, you stay active. And when you're active, you are less likely to be hanging out in the kitchen.

FLUSH FLASH

Before beginning this or any other exercise program, please consult your physician.

I'm a forty-three-year-old woman, who has always been looking toward better health. But through life's many transitions, I have found myself depressed, unfocused, bloated, and eventually gaining 10 pounds on my once toned body frame. Lately, I've been exhausted, tired, and lacking any motivation to do regular activities or even pursue anything new.

Fat Flush came at a critical time when I needed to shift from what was becoming an unhealthy cycle. Exercise has always been in my regimen, but that alone wasn't working, so I started your program. I notice a huge, huge difference! I've lost weight, gained energy, an am much more alert.

—SUZANN PROKOSCH

Phase 1 Exercise Program

GOAL: WORKING THE LYMPHATICS

✓ **Warm-ups and stretching.** Whenever you're going to exercise—even if it is just going for a walk—be sure to always begin your session by warming up your muscles for five to ten minutes by marching in place and swinging your arms back and forth. Then spend five to ten minutes gently stretching your muscles, ligaments, and tendons to improve flexibility and prevent potential injury, muscle strains, and stiffness. Stretch your arms, your legs, your inner thighs, etc., by holding each stretch pose for fifteen seconds and building up to a minute as you gain more flexibility.

✓ **Bouncing off fat.** As you learned in Chapter 2, purifying the lymphatic system is vital for ridding your body of cellulite-like deposits during phase 1 of the Fat Flush. Since it doesn't have a pump like the heart, the lymphatic system has to be exercised, relying on muscle contractions for its flow via the thighs and arms. The best way to do this—to give those fatty deposits the old heave-ho—is by cleansing your lymphatic system either with a bouncing action or by moving your arms while walking briskly.

To give your lymphatic drainage system a complete cellular cleansing during all phases of Fat Flush, I'd like you to consider purchasing a minitrampoline (or small rebounder) (see Chapter 12). These units typically stand 8 inches from the floor and are anywhere from 36 to 40 inches in diameter. You'll bounce on it every day for five minutes to gently ease waste materials out of the lymphatic system. The greatest thing about this lymph-cleansing exercise is that virtually anyone can do it, regardless of age or certain physical challenges. Individuals who can't walk can still benefit from this exercise by sitting on the rebounder while someone else bounces on it.

Use of a minitrampoline (or rebounder) has proven to be an efficient form of exercise with virtually no harmful side effects. Your cardiovascular fitness will excel, and you will be toning your body at the same time. It fires up cellular metabolism, energizing every cell with fresh oxygen and nutrients. The low impact (such as the light pressure on the thighs) stimulates drainage, easing waste material out of the lymphatic system. In approximately two weeks, you should notice that your legs, buttocks, and ankles are becoming toned and those orange peel–like cellulite deposits are smoothing out.

You can help improve your lymph flow by (1) breathing deeply through your nose, letting oxygen into the lower part of your lungs, (2) not sitting for extended periods, which restricts lymphatic flow in your thoracic cavity, and (3) not overdoing your exercise routine, which augments oxidative stress.

And I think you'll find bouncing to be a lot of fun. The great thing about it is that you can do it anywhere you live—an apartment or home, and you can even take it outside.

BOUNCING TIPS

✓ **Clothing**
No special clothing is required. Select comfortable apparel that won't interfere with your bouncing routine or get caught in the unit.

✓ **Feet**
Bounce barefoot for freer movements and control. Avoid wearing socks, nylons, or slippery shoes or slippers. If you must wear shoes, choose rubber, nonskid soles.

✓ **Technique**
Strive for 100 jumping jacks (approximately five minutes). With legs together and arms down at your sides, leap up. As you come back down to the trampoline, spread your legs and throw your arms above your head. Keeping that position, jump up again—but this time when you come down, go back to your beginning position of legs together and hands to your sides.

✓ **Placement**
Keep your minitrampoline handy so you'll be encouraged to use it. Bounce in a well-lit area. Exercising in front of a mirror is a good way to perfect your technique.

Walking for health. The next part of your phase 1 exercise regimen is a twenty-minute brisk walk, which I would like you to get into the habit of doing every day or at least five times per week. Walk briskly with your arms swinging along your sides in sync with your pace to keep the lymphatic system moving. Distance is not important—your time, however, is.

An aerobic exercise, brisk walking keeps your heart and lungs strong, promoting cardiovascular health, energy, endurance, and the production of endorphins. As a matter of fact, the United States and Japan released studies demonstrating that individuals who walked habitually had two times the reduction in mortality rate and complications related to coronary artery disease of their more sedentary counterparts.

During this gentle Fat Flush phase, I do not want you using your energy reserves for strenuous movement. This is why it is a good idea to monitor the intensity of your workout. You can do this a number of ways.

An easy method is to pace yourself, walking approximately 1 to 1.5 miles in twenty minutes. Walking any quicker stimulates additional oxidative stress. Breathe deeply and regularly through your nose during your workout to help reduce potential damage from free radicals.

You may even want to try a more technical approach, which I will strongly encourage in phase 3. What you do is track your pulse rate while exercising to ensure that the intensity of your workout falls within certain zones of your maximum heart rate, called *max HR.*

You can do this quite easily by first figuring your max HR, which requires nothing more than subtracting your age from 220. For instance, if you are 32 years old, your max HR would be 188 beats per minute.

For phase 1 of your Fat Flush exercise program, I recommend keeping your heart rate at 50 percent of your max HR or slightly above. Thus, if your max HR is 188 beats per minute, then 50 percent of this number would equal a heart rate of 94. (If you don't want to do the math, look

WALKING TIPS

✓ **Clothing**

- In warmer weather, choose lightweight materials that absorb perspiration easily and dry quickly.
- In colder weather, wear loose, layered clothing made of natural material. Avoid plastic fabrics or polyester, since they don't let your skin breathe—especially important for menopausal women. Keep your head and neck covered in inclement weather.
- In rainy weather, try to stay dry by wearing waterproof garments.

✓ **Shoes**

- Wear comfortable shoes with firm heels and supportive arches. Choose shoes with breathable upper material and thick, flexible soles. Be sure you have sufficient toe area with soft padding.

✓ **Water**

- Drink plenty of water before, during, and after your workout to avoid dehydration. You can even drink more than your daily requirement. In warm weather or dry climates, drink sufficient water before you begin exercising to replace what will be lost in perspiration.

✓ **Posture**

- Walk upright with your shoulders relaxed. Swing your arms at your side. Step from your heel to your toe.

up your age on the table below. Column 2 shows your max HR; columns 3, 4, and 5 show the pulse rates for the 50, 60, and 70 percent zones. Use the number in column 3, the 50 percent zone, for phase 1 of the exercise plan.)

How can you tell your heart rate? Just check your pulse rate while exercising. You can either use a heart rate monitor strapped around your chest or feel your pulse rate via your radial artery (on the underside of your wrist). Place your index and middle fingers on the thumb side of your wrist. Determine your heart rate (beats per minute) by counting the beats for thirty seconds and multiplying that number by 2. (A quicker but less accurate method is to take your pulse for six seconds and then add a zero after that number. For example, 14 beats + 0 = 140.)

Keeping within the 50 and 60 percent zones is especially good for walking or for individuals who are breaking into an exercise program for the first time, even though it isn't intense enough to reap broader cardiovascular benefits. Also, exercising within these zones has demonstrated an ability to reduce body fat, cholesterol, and blood pressure levels and lessen the potential for strains, injuries, and degenerative disease. At this intensity level, 85 percent of the calories you burn are fat, 10 percent are carbohydrate, and 5 percent are protein.

ASSESSING YOUR HEART RATE

AGE, YEARS	MAXIMUM HEART RATE, BEATS PER MINUTE	TARGET HEART RATE, BEATS PER MINUTE		
		50 PERCENT	60 PERCENT	70 PERCENT
15–19	201	100	121	140
20–24	196	98	118	137
25–29	191	96	115	133
30–34	186	93	112	130
35–39	181	91	109	126
40–44	176	88	106	123
45-49	171	86	103	120
50–54	166	83	100	116
55–59	161	81	97	113
60–64	156	78	94	109
65–69	151	76	91	106
70–74	146	73	88	102
75–80	141	71	85	99

Rule of thumb: Whatever your target heart rate, you should exercise only at a level that lets you breathe and move comfortably—and that is safe for your body.

When you actually take your walk is entirely up to you. However, mornings before breakfast seem to be the best fat-burning choice for most of us. Before breakfast, the level of glycogen (carbohydrate storage of fuel in the liver) runs low, causing your body to choose fat instead for its energy. As it is busy using up these stored fatty acids, your body becomes a fat-eating machine.

Cool-down. Just as warming up and stretching are critical before beginning your workout session, taking five to ten minutes to cool down is equally important in finishing your routine. It gives your body a chance to gently wind down, causing blood flow to return to normal.

PHASE 1 FAT FLUSH EXERCISE WRAP-UP

Warm-Up and Stretching	At least 5 minutes, every session
Bouncing	5 minutes, daily
Brisk Walking	20 minutes, 5–7 times a week
Cool-Down	At least 5 minutes, every session

I was on the program for a few days when I noticed the cellulite lumps on my upper arms had noticeably diminished! Now I can see those triceps I've been exercising so hard.

—Ann V. Leigh

The Fat Flush Plan has worked a true miracle on me. I'm twenty-eight and quite overweight. I sit behind a computer under fluorescent lights all day. I lost 16 pounds, my skin cleared up, my eyes are brighter, and my hair looks better than it's looked in a while.

—Georgia Anna Rodriguez

Phase 2 Exercise Program

GOAL: BUILDING ENDURANCE

During this phase of your Fat Flush Plan, you will continue your phase 1 exercise routine—but add another ten minutes to your brisk walking time.

If you are keeping tabs on your heart rate, you may want to try upping your exercise intensity slightly, to 60 percent of your max HR. Using the preceding example, if your max HR is 188 beats per minute, your pulse rate while exercising would be 60 percent of that, or 112 beats per minute.

Working within this zone helps your body to access stored fat for energy. As a result, you will burn more calories while at the same time helping your cardiovascular system become more fit. Approximately 85 percent of the calories you burn will be fat, with 10 percent carbohydrates and 5 percent protein.

PHASE 2 FAT FLUSH EXERCISE WRAP-UP

Warm-Up and Stretching	At least 5 minutes every session
Bouncing	5 minutes, daily
Brisk Walking	30 minutes, 5–7 times a week
Cool-Down	At least 5 minutes, every session

I have followed the Fat Flush Plan with great success! I don't know how much weight I've lost—I don't weigh myself—but I now have great muscle definition, more energy, and skin that is getting more radiant every day. Thank you!

—KATIE MARR

Phase 3 Exercise Program

GOAL: STRENGTHENING MUSCLE MASS

Now that you have graduated to the lifestyle phase of the Fat Flush Plan, you are ready to build on your phase 1 and 2 foundation. The endurance you have developed over the last several weeks, along with the added fuel from the foods you are reintroducing, lays the groundwork for expanding your exercise regimen.

Your brisk walk also will extend ten minutes, to a total of forty minutes five times a week. And if you haven't already been doing it, now is the time to watch your target heart rate for the entire walk.

Try to move up to 70 percent of your max HR (the figure in the last column of the heart rate table). Training at 70 percent or slightly higher (to 80 percent) puts you in the aerobic zone, where half your burned calories are from fat, almost half are from carbohydrates, and less than 1 percent are from protein. In this zone, your blood vessel size and number rise as your cardiovascular and respiratory systems improve.

You'll also be topping off your lifestyle regimen with a new exercise to tone and sculpt your body: weight training.

Weight training. I am not talking about Herculean strength. Even using 2- to 5-pound dumbbells can help you build lean muscle mass. And remember, muscle accelerates metabolism and burns calories longer, even while you sleep.

Maintaining lean muscle mass is especially important for women, because we tend to lose ¼ to ⅓ pound of muscle every year past age thirty-five. And if you're a woman who is thinking that you'll soon have Mr. America–type arms, don't. High testosterone levels are responsible for those muscular physiques. Since women don't have to contend with that type of hormonal level, weight training actually will help to improve the tone and strength of your muscles as well as strengthen your musculoskeletal system.

You should weight train at least twice a week or every other day. Start out by following a regimen created by a professional. You don't have to sign up for a personal trainer; you could rent a video or go to the library. You might even get help from a local health gym.

Weight-training routines tend to isolate certain muscle groups. Typically, your workout would focus on different groups at least once a week. You may want to consider varying your routine over time to work your muscles differently.

If you start with lower weights (2 to 5 pounds), you will have to do more repetitions than if you were already lifting 10-pound weights (your goal). As you increase your muscle mass—and fat-burning potential—your actual weight may not budge a whole lot, because muscle weighs more than fat. This is okay, because you are reducing body fat, which is your goal. Studies reveal that weight-training women generally add 3 to 5 pounds of muscle and lose the same amount of fat pounds. Quite often women drop one or two dress sizes, thanks to their more toned bodies.

WEIGHT TRAINING TIPS

✓ **Clothing**

- Choose apparel that doesn't impede movement. Dress for the room temperature.

✓ **Shoes**

- Wear comfortable shoes with good traction.

✓ **Water**

- Drink plenty of water before, during, and after your workout to avoid dehydration. Feel free to drink more than your alloted 48 ounces of plain water on phase 3 for this purpose. In warm weather or dry climates, drink sufficient water before you begin exercising to replace what will be lost in perspiration. Generally, figure on drinking a quart of water per 100 pounds of body weight.

✓ **Routine**

- Follow a program designed by a certified expert.
- Work different muscles on different days, taking a day off in between. Try working your chest, shoulders, and biceps one time, then your triceps and back two days later. Then, two days after that, target your lower body.
- Keep your back straight while lifting.
- Lift weights slowly with proper form.
- Breathe out when you lift and breathe naturally to keep muscles oxidized. Avoid holding your breath as you lift, since it hinders the flow of blood in and out of the brain.
- Take three or four seconds to lift the weights and even longer to lower them.
- Start with lighter weights, increasing poundage by either 1-pound, 2-pound, or 5-pound increments each workout to a total of 10-pound weights.

Double your fat-burning power. Lifting weights uses glycogen for energy. Thus, after you're done using your weights, it would be a good time to do some aerobic exercise to burn even more fat—such as taking a brisk walk. The aerobic activity causes your body (now low in glycogen from lifting weights) to use fatty acids for fuel, similar to how it reacts to exercise before breakfast.

You may want to consider moving your combination weight training and brisk walk to later in the afternoon to accelerate calorie loss another notch. Apparently our muscles and joints tend to be more limber between 3 and 5 P.M., which is the same time our airways are more open and we breathe easier. This combination causes us to feel good and actually burn through a higher amount of calories per minute—with less effort.

PHASE 3 FAT FLUSH EXERCISE WRAP-UP

Warm-Up and Stretching	At least 5 minutes every session
Bouncing	5 minutes, daily
Brisk Walking	40 minutes, 5 times a week
Weight Training	10–15 minutes at least twice a week or every other day
Cool-Down	At least 5 minutes, every session

SLEEP

You may not think of sleep as a key component of weight loss, but it definitely is. Our bodies run on a biological clock. Every cell is tuned in to this clock, relying on it for its metabolic processes, such as your hormone levels, blood sugar levels, metabolic rates, sodium/potassium levels, and even your body temperature and immune functions—many of the same concerns you have been reading about throughout this book that affect your weight.

Getting to bed and rising at specific times are vital to the success of these body functions. If your lifestyle isn't in sync with your biological clock, your health, well-being, and (believe it or not) weight loss goals suffer. What happens is that your internal sensors go awry, which actually can cause you to overeat. According to statistics, poor sleepers consume approximately 15 percent more food than their sleep-nourished counterparts. Without proper sleep, they often feel tired and grab high-carbohydrate "comfort" foods that are also high in sugar to boost energy. Their bodies also begin to store fat, taking the fatigue as a signal that a crisis is approaching.

When you get a restful, deep sleep, energy levels are restored and hormones are reset. However, poor sleep does more than cause a drop in your energy level—it also creates problems with your hormones. In fact, University of Chicago researchers say that lack of sleep could even make you flabby. Some scientists believe that the poor sleep impedes surges of growth hormone that is needed to promote lean muscle tissue and reduce body fat, resulting in a deficiency.

Compounding the problem, insufficient sleep forces your cortisol level to rise. As you learned in Chapter 2, cortisol works in concert with other chemicals to quicken fat storage, targeting the central fat cells. It releases glucose and fatty acids so that muscles have energy—and consequently stimulates your appetite to encourage you to replenish fuel. When your twenty-first-century lifestyle causes you to become sleep-deprived (thanks to crazy work schedules, juggling two jobs, getting a degree, and managing a family), your cortisol level stays elevated. As a result, you may find yourself wanting to grab a late-night snack, such as some sugary food, that only aggravates the situation by promoting even more cortisol production.

For most of us Americans, this spells trouble, because we have embraced a new twenty-four-hour mentality. We are busy around the clock nowadays—spending more time shopping at all-night convenience stores, grocery markets, or national-chain superstores. And, of course, there is the Internet. We do our banking, take courses, make travel arrangements, search an infinite number of topics, chitchat with friends, read newspapers, etc., to the wee hours of the morning now that we can be online anytime, anywhere.

Keeping this in mind, these recent statistics should come as no surprise: According to a 2001 "Sleep in America" poll conducted by the National Sleep Foundation (NSF), a large sector of our population is deprived of sleep. The NSF, which examines the connection between Americans' lifestyles, sleep habits, and sleep problems, discovered that 63 percent of adults do not get eight hours of sleep, the recommended amount for good health and top performance. Practically one-third of us get even less than seven hours of sleep on weeknights. With our twenty-first-century lifestyles, it is no wonder that as much as one-third of the population reports getting even less sleep than just five years ago. And 69 percent of us often have to contend with sleep problems in one form or another.

It is a vicious cycle that strikes a familiar chord, especially in women, who tend to suffer the most. Their sleeping habits are often affected by hormonal changes, menses, the advent of children, and stress from family and work. Joyce A. Walsleben, Ph.D., director of the Sleep Disorders Center at the New York University School of Medicine, says that "women are probably the most sleep-deprived creatures on earth. . . . the average woman aged thirty to sixty sleeps only six hours and forty-one minutes during the workweek. . . . Most people need at least eight hours of sleep to function at their best."

Fat Flush Sleep Program

It is really quite simple. You will follow your internal biological clock, in sync with your daily rhythm of cortisol. This means going to bed by that magical hour of 10 P.M., when your cortisol levels diminish to their lowest levels, three hours after sunset. And you'll rise when your cortisol levels peak in the early morning, a refreshing eight hours later.

Understandably, you may have times when your hectic day makes it difficult to unwind. Here are some bedtime tips you may find helpful to protect your beauty rest:

Sleep tips

AVOID:

Eating two hours before bedtime.
Taking a nap after 4 P.M. or for over an hour.
Exercising too close to bedtime.
Lying in bed awake. Instead, try reading, putting on some music, watching TV, etc., until you can fall asleep.
Maintaining extreme temperatures in your bedroom.

TRY:

Sleeping in a cooler room, between 60 and 65°F. A warm room impedes sleep and causes more awakenings. Use a fan or air-conditioner to keep you cool and comfortable.
Keeping your bedtime peaceful and your bedroom for sleep-related activities only.
Making sure that you have a comfortable bed to sleep on.
Getting to bed and waking up the same time every day.
Waking up with the sun, if possible, to reset your internal biological clock daily. Getting an hour of morning sunlight (or using extremely bright lights in the morning) could help with falling asleep at night.
Taking a warm bath. Researchers suggest that taking a fifteen-minute bath of 105°F approximately ninety minutes before going to bed is helpful. The rise in body temperature, followed by the decline in the core temperature, signals the body that it's bedtime.

JOURNALING

As I have previously encouraged you to do, the best way to keep tabs on yourself throughout your Fat Flush journey is to keep a journal. Hands down, journaling has proven to be a helpful factor in attaining weight loss goals. This certainly was the case for participants in a research study conducted by the National Weight Control Registry. These individuals, who had to lose more than 30 pounds and maintain the loss for one year at minimum in order to take part in the study, found that keeping a diet journal proved elemental to their success.

Their achievement might very well be linked to the fact that journaling creates the perfect place to discover what motivates your food desires, what triggers those cravings, and what's really going on beneath those surface feelings. By taking the time to write these things down, you'll reduce anxiety and stay in touch with yourself. Stress researcher Ann McGee-Cooper, Ed.D., suggests that by writing through emotions, you actually may be less likely to fall prey to stress. And since stress can lead to weight gain, journaling through those feelings could keep you from abandoning your weight and fitness objectives. Additional recent studies support this fact, indicating that fifteen minutes of journaling each day can cut stress levels and even bolster the immune system by 76 percent.

So, if a coworker gets you steamed up, grab your Fat Flush journal, not those doughnuts. By the time you write through it, you'll feel the stress ease away and that desire for junk food fade.

Besides tracking meals, supplements, exercise, and sleep and helping you through stressful times, journaling provides numerous other opportunities for insight. You can jot down personal concerns, note changes in your health and emotions, trace the origins of specific food reactions as you reintroduce quality carbohydrates and dairy into your diet, and even find something you did each day to deserve a personal pat on the back. Most important, journaling will help you learn more about and connect with the most important person in your life—you.

Journaling Basics

The primary tenet of journaling centers on that tried-and-true adage "Honesty is the best policy." So don't be timid. Jot down whatever words and thoughts come to mind, recording everything and anything. For instance, if you're hungry, write it down. It's not a crime. In fact, it is a rather typical response as you get started on phase 1.

And this holds true for other responses as well, such as your sinuses draining, your digestive system getting a bit upset, or your skin breaking out. Don't fret over these things. Just write them all down because these side effects are actually good signs—and not at all unusual. They mean that your body is cleansing itself and Fat Flush is working!

Journaling will be of special help as you begin to add back other foods (in phases 2 and 3). It's not uncommon for some people to notice food reactions, such as gas, bloating, sleepiness, headaches, or cramps, which can occur anywhere from ten minutes to twelve hours after you've eaten. By honestly tracking these types of responses, you'll be able to clearly identify which foods are hidden sources of weight gain and take control of your weight loss goals.

When you journal is really up to you. Some Fat Flushers like to write things down as they occur, so they carry their journals with them throughout the day. You might want to find a few moments at the end of the day if you can properly recall what you ate, etc. *You determine what will work best for your lifestyle.*

Regardless of when you journal, the most important thing you can do is be kind to yourself. Don't be critical. Go back every few days and read what you wrote and how you were feeling. This will help you learn who you are and identify positive trends you may otherwise be missing. It also will help you learn to become your own best friend.

How to Create Your Fat Flush Journal

There are several ways to get started. You can use a notebook, pick up an inexpensive journal book with blank pages at your local bookstore, or create your own journal pages on a computer to print out and insert in a nicely colored project folder.

There are ten categories that I think would be especially helpful to have in your daily Fat Flush journal. However, please feel free to pick and choose whichever areas mean the most to you. I've given you a sample page from one of my Fat Flushers at the end of the chapter to give you an idea of how your journal could look. Be sure to leave yourself enough room in each category, particularly the ones where you may be inclined to write more. And always date every page for accurate referencing. There are some blank journal pages provided in the Appendix for you to photocopy and use if you wish.

Here are some areas and categories that have worked for Fat Flushers in the past:

✓ PHASES. At the top of each journal page, title it according to the Fat Flush phase you're in: "Accelerating Weight Loss," "Ongoing Weight Loss," or "Lifestyle."

✓ GOALS. Determine a goal for each phase of your Fat Flush journey. Maybe you want to drop 3 to 6 inches off your hips, fit into that favorite outfit hanging in the back of your closet, or get rid of that ugly cellulite on your thighs and buttocks. Decide what is most important to you at each phase.

Set your Fat Flush goal, visualize it, and then follow the program with your goal in front of you. Based on my experience of working with thousands of individuals, those who set goals enjoy a number of benefits. They appear to be more contented with their performances and actually perform better. Goal-oriented people also appear more self-confident, tend to worry less, and display better concentration.

Reality check: Be good to yourself by setting realistic goals. A 40-year-old can't expect to look 25 again. Set goals that are attainable for your age, stage of life, and body frame. Here are two helpful charts to determine the average weight for both women and men.

FOR WOMEN			
Aged 25 to 59 years Weight in pounds, per frame type (with indoor clothing weighing 3 pounds and wearing 1-inch-heeled shoes)			
HEIGHT	SMALL FRAME	MEDIUM FRAME	LARGE FRAME
4′ 10″	102–111	109–121	118–131
4′ 11″	103–113	111–123	120–134
5′ 0″	104–115	113–126	122–137
5′ 1″	106–118	115–129	125–140
5′ 2″	108–121	118–132	128–143
5′ 3″	111–124	121–135	131–147
5′ 4″	114–127	124–138	134–151
5′ 5″	117–130	127–141	137–155
5′ 6″	120–133	130–144	140–159
5′ 7″	123–136	133–147	143–163
5′ 8″	126–139	136–150	146–167
5′ 9″	129–142	139–153	149–170
5′ 10″	132–145	142–156	152–173
5′ 11″	135–148	145–159	155–176
6′ 0″	138–151	148–162	158–179

FOR MEN			
Aged 25 to 59 years Weight in pounds, per frame type (with indoor clothing weighing 3 pounds and wearing 1-inch-heeled shoes)			
HEIGHT	SMALL FRAME	MEDIUM FRAME	LARGE FRAME
5′ 2″	128–134	131–141	138–150
5′ 3″	130–136	133–143	140–153
5′ 4″	132–138	135–145	142–156
5′ 5″	134–140	137–148	144–160
5′ 6″	136–142	139–151	146–164
5′ 7″	138–145	142–154	149–168
5′ 8″	140–148	145–157	152–172
5′ 9″	142–151	148–160	155–176
5′ 10″	144–154	151–163	158–180
5′ 11″	146–157	154–166	161–184
6′ 0″	149–160	157–170	164–188
6′ 1″	152–164	160–174	168–192
6′ 2″	155–168	164–178	172–197
6′ 3″	158–172	167–182	176–202
6′ 4″	162–176	171–187	181–207

- ✓ **REWARDS.** Your dedicated efforts deserve recognition, so you may want to think of a way to reward yourself for reaching the goal of each phase. Choose something you would really look forward to, such as treating yourself to a spa manicure and pedicure, buying some new clothes, or doing something special. You might even want to schedule time in that busy day planner of yours to soak in a relaxing bubble bath with lighted candles and soothing music.
- ✓ **MEALS, BEVERAGES, AND SNACKS.** Jot down everything you eat, from the Long Life Cocktail and hot water with lemon juice to every snack and meal. Tracking your food gives you good cause to adopt the "mindful eating" approach. Instead of eating on the run or eating while doing something else—such as watching TV or reading a book—focus on your meal. Set the table, making it and your meal visually appealing. Take the time to chew the food, savoring every bite. By staying "in the now" when you eat, you'll be less likely to overeat because you'll recognize when you are full instead of mindlessly munching on more helpings. If you stay aware of your eating, you also will be able to discern why you are eating in the first place. Is it emotional or physical? Identifying the reason and writing it down empowers you to finally address the reason behind your hunger.
- ✓ **SUPPLEMENTS.** Keep track of what you're taking and how much. Did you remember to take your multiple vitamin? Gamma-linolenic acid (GLA)? Fat-burner?
- ✓ **WEEKLY MEASUREMENTS.** Once a week, measure your chest, waist, hips, and thighs. Some Fat Flushers like to measure their arms, above the elbows. Remember, losing inches is the key to a slimmer you, not pounds on a scale. Inch loss reveals true fat loss, a real assessment of your progress. The scale will tend to move up and down occasionally for other reasons—such as having your period, for example.

If you're a stickler for accuracy, you may want to also assess your body mass index (BMI), which is used to determine how much fat you are carrying. This simple assessment helps you determine whether you're at an ideal weight, overweight, or dealing with obesity. Although the BMI is a useful tool, it can overestimate the fat percentage in more athletic or muscular individuals. I also wouldn't suggest calculating the BMI of children or adolescents. To determine body fat, your BMI is calculated like this:

1. Multiply your weight in pounds by 0.45.
2. Multiply your height in inches by 0.025.
3. Take your answer from step 2 and square it (multiply it by itself).
4. Divide your answer from step 1 by your answer from step 3.

The result is your BMI. For example, let's say you weigh 175 pounds and are 5 feet, 6 inches tall. Then

1. Multiply 175 (your weight) by 0.45: 175 x 0.45 = 78.75.
2. Convert 5 feet, 6 inches (your height) into inches: 5 x 12 = 60 +6 = 66 inches. Now multiply 66 by 0.025: 66 x 0.025 = 1.65.

3. Square your final answer in step 2 by multiplying the number by itself: 1.65 times 1.65 = 2.72.
4. Divide 78.75 (your answer in step 1) by 2.72 (your answer in step 3) to get your BMI: 78.75 ÷ 2.72 = 28.95.

According to the 1998 federal Obesity Clinical Guidelines, a BMI between 25 and 29.9 is considered overweight. Anything greater than this (30 and over) is labeled obesity. If your BMI is 25 or higher, you are not alone. Approximately 114 million adults in this country fall into this category. A BMI between 19 and 24 is ideal, whereas a BMI below 19 may indicate that an individual is underweight.

✓ FOOD FOR THOUGHT. Jot down whatever is going on with you that is food-related. For instance, did you spend the afternoon with food on the brain? Have you noticed your cravings fading away? Did you notice yourself feeling drowsy or tired after adding carbs (in phase 2) or dairy (in phase 3)? Are you experiencing sugar or caffeine withdrawal? Did you slip off the Fat Flush wagon?

✓ HEALTH AND WELLNESS NOTES. Are your menses more regular? Is your skin clearing up and looking more radiant? Are your bowel movements regular? How are you feeling—more calm, less anxious, more energetic? Have your mood swings evened out?

✓ EXERCISE ROUTINE. How many minutes did you walk, or do the suggested trampoline workout, or spend on strength training (required in phase 3)? How did you feel during and after your exercise session? Is it getting easier each time?

✓ SLEEP TIME. Are you making it to bed by 10 P.M. and getting your eight hours of sleep in?

✓ REFLECTIONS. This is the place to go when you feel like venting or talking something through, whether it's about work, your family, your weight loss, a desire to snack, etc. Use this area to jot it all down, thinking of it as your own personal sounding board—a place you can go to that is safe. No one is going to criticize you here. Then look back on it a few days later. It's a good way to learn more about who you are and what makes you tick—and what ticks you off!

✓ DAILY ACKNOWLEDGMENT. Even if you didn't do 100 percent today, reflect on what you did do and acknowledge something good about yourself. Bolster your self-esteem and keep your momentum going by patting yourself on the back for whatever positive thing you discovered. Write down, "Today I did this well: ________________," and fill in the blank. Recognize it as a good step, however small. After all, it's the little steps that lead us to those great accomplishments.

FAT FLUSH JOURNAL

PHASE 1

MY PHASE I GOAL: *Drop 6 pounds so I can wear my favorite blue jeans again.*

MY PHASE I REWARD: *Get a spa pedicure at the new salon in town.*

TODAY'S DATE: *August 15*

Meals, Beverages, & Snacks

- UPON RISING – *Had my Long Life Cocktail*
- BEFORE BREAKFAST – *Drank my 8 oz of hot water and lemon*
- BREAKFAST – *Made a Blueberry Smoothie*
- MIDMORNING SNACK – *Hard-boiled egg*
- BEFORE LUNCH – *Had 8-oz of cran-water*
- LUNCH – *Brought my beef stir fry to work: 4 ounces lean beef with bok choy, mushrooms, bean sprouts. Added ginger and a bit of cayenne for flavor. Also made a red-leaf salad with a few radishes, celery, fresh parsley, and some cukes. Used 1 tablespoon of flaxseed oil for dressing. Also drank 8 oz of cran-water.*
- MID-AFTERNOON SNACK – *Drank 2 glasses of cran-water (8-oz each)*
- 4 P.M. SNACK – *Had 1 pear*
- BEFORE DINNER - *Had 8-oz of cran-water*
- DINNER – *Made the cumin & cinnamon-scented Eggplant Delight with a side of yellow squash, asparagus, some fresh cilantro, and water chestnuts. Sauteed some greens in veggie broth with a bit of garlic.*
- MIDEVENING – *Had my Long Life Cocktail*

Supplements

Took my GLA-90 capsules (2 w/breakfast & 2 w/dinner). Had mymulti and mineral supp w/breakfast and dinner. Took my Weight Loss formula at each meal.

Measurements

- BUST/CHEST *36 inches*
- WAIST *27 inches*
- HIPS *38 inches*
- THIGHS *22 inches*

FOOD FOR THOUGHT – *During my afternoon break with Sally and the gang, someone brought our usual Friday "snack"—a coconut cream Marie Callender pie! That was tough to turn down, but I actually felt satisfied once I had my Fat Flush snack.*

HEALTH & WELLNESS NOTES – *My skin is looking better than it ever has—even my husband noticed how good it looks. And I've got more energy today. I used to feel drowsy by mid-afternoon, but I actually whizzed through it with energy to spare!*

EXERCISE – *Went for my morning walk after I got up. It 's getting easier and my mind feels clear and ready for the day.*

SLEEP TIME – *Got to bed a little after 10 pm. Now that I've got the temperature cooler, I'm finding it easier to sleep straight through my 8 hours.*

REFLECTIONS – *Had an argument with a co-worker, who was trying to muscle in on my area to make herself look good.*

I got so upset and walked out of the office down to the vending machine. Felt so much like grabbing some cookies and a candy bar, but then decided to step outside and walk it off for a few minutes. Glad I did. It helped relieve the anger a bit and gave me time to regroup and not blow my diet with sugar!

DAILY ACKNOWLEDGMENT – *Today I avoided the temptation of eating my usual sugar snacks twice—and that is a great thing! Yeah me!*

INSIDER TIP | Fat Flush Journal pages that you can photocopy and use are provided in the Appendix.

CHAPTER

8 The Fat Flush Plan Away from Home

Of all the medicine created out of the Earth, food is the chief.

—SIR ROBERT MCCARRISON, M.D.

If there is one thing I have learned over the years, it is that fast foods are here to stay. Eating away from home has become a way of life in our twenty-first century. America is host to nearly 170,000 fast-food establishments and 3 million vending machines that sell soft drinks. And at least 50 percent of our food budget is spent on both food and drink eaten outside the home. Thus, it is no wonder that the food industry shells out nearly $11 billion on promotions per year. McDonald's alone spent over a billion dollars in 1998. The soft drink pushers spent $115.5 million. All of this "helps ensure that Americans are not more than a few steps from immediate sources of relatively nonnutritious food," according to *Public Health Reports* of January–February 2000.

Yet, with a little bit of know-how, you can easily Fat Flush your way through the fast-food lane. You just need a basic road map to help you make the best food decisions. And the road map I'm talking about is far from complicated—it is quite simple, in fact. It is built on the absolutely best Fat Flushing foods, based on the foundational principles of the right protein, friendly carbohydrates, and fat-burning fats. Thus, you will enjoy meals that are built on such staples as eggs, lean red meat, fish, vegetables, salads, fruit, and even a little bit of butter. Fortunately, many of these foods can be found just about anywhere these days.

Convenience, however, carries a definite price. You can blow a whole day's worth of salt and calories in a single fast-food meal if you are not careful. Thus, there is some challenge in making the Fat Flush Plan work at a fast-food restaurant. On the other hand, many fast-food places offer healthier options these days, such as rotisserie-prepared chicken and turkey, featured as home-style meals.

Because of the greater variety of foods available on Lifestyle, it is much easier to eat out when in phase 3 than when in the first two Fat Flush phases. You can enjoy Fat Flushing meals away from home if you avoid certain food items, make some savvy substitutions, lighten up on the food combination rules, and remember to take your flaxseed oil or flaxseed dressing with you—in those little film canisters mentioned in Chapter 4 so that it is protected from heat, air, and light.

ON THE ROAD WHILE FAT FLUSHING

Whether it is fast foods or fine dining, the food choices you make can either boost fat burning or create fat storage. It is really up to you.

By far one of the biggest challenges to eating out is avoiding the trans-fat traps. These fats include the liver-clogging, weight control–inhibiting hydrogenated oils, processed oils, margarine, and fried foods. These oils, as discussed previously, should be strictly avoided because of the trans-fatty acids they contain. The more common foods that contain them—which you wouldn't even consider on the Fat Flush Plan anyway—include fast-food biscuits, Danish pastries, chocolate chip cookies, muffins, french fries, fried onion rings, processed cheese, mayonnaise, tartar sauce, and chicken nuggets. They are virtually everywhere!

You will recall that while no one knows for certain how much trans fat the body can tolerate, many experts feel that the daily intake should not exceed 2 g. The problem is that the most popular fast foods are really top-heavy with those nasty trans fats. In fact, the *New York Times* reported that nutritional expert Mary Enig, Ph.D. found an incredible "8 g of trans-fatty acids in a large order of french fries cooked in partially hydrogenated vegetable oil, 10 g in a typical serving of fast-food fried chicken or fried fish, and 8 g in 2 ounces of imitation cheese."

Just remember that the trans fats I want you to avoid, as well as the saturated ones that you want to minimize, may be lurking in creamy cheese sauces and dressings, which also are loaded with plenty of regular salt and sugar. This is why I encourage you to "lemonize" your salad by simply squeezing a lemon (or lime) over it instead of a restaurant dressing, if you haven't brought your own.

As a rule of thumb, if you are on phase 3 of the plan (Lifestyle Fat Flush), choose sauces that are based on wine (the alcohol burns off in cooking) or lemon over the creamed ones. Or opt for a light marinara rather than a heavy-duty cheese and tomato sauce. Likewise, do not make a daily habit of eating cream soups. Go for the vegetable- or tomato-based ones so that you won't be overloading on certain fats. And remember that on the Lifestyle Fat Flush, you also can enjoy bean soup as part of your daily quality carbs—exercising moderation, of course.

You also will want to hold back on mayonnaise (although a tablespoon *is* allowed on Lifestyle), because most commercially prepared mayonnaise products are made with partially hydrogenated soybean oil. So there goes ordering those tuna, egg, shrimp, and chicken salads, as well as coleslaw and potato salad (even for Lifestyle Fat Flushers), because they all contain mayonnaise. At home, you can use a brand such as

Spectrum, which is made with nonhydrogenated, trans-fat-free soybean oil. Think in terms of mustard or even yogurt instead of commercial mayonnaise. A side of salsa, guacamole, or hummus (chickpea paste made with sesame for Lifestyle Fat Flushers) cut with lemon juice or fresh lemons can really satisfy your tastebuds. And they don't contain the trans-fat factors like mayonnaise-based dips.

GOING AGAINST THE GRAIN

When it comes to bread, muffins, crackers, and rolls, try to eliminate those made with refined white flour. However, this will be next to impossible in most fast-food establishments. By the way, this also goes for pasta, especially when it is the focus of your meal. No matter what the glamorous incarnation (e.g., penne, angel hair, ziti, spaghetti, or macaroni), pasta is almost always made from white flour—that simple carbohydrate that is rapidly absorbed into your bloodstream and sends glucose and then fat-promoting insulin levels soaring. A better bet, whenever possible, is to order whole-grain food items, such as brown rice. And do remember that like pasta, even sourdough—which may have some redeeming qualities—is still made with white refined flour.

FATS OF LIFE

Since not all fats are considered off-limits on the Fat Flush Plan and some are actually good for you, be sure to choose foods that feature healthy fats. Olive and sesame oils are the oils of choice for Lifestyle Fat Flush enjoyment. They are readily available in many specialty restaurants, especially Italian, Greek, Spanish, Chinese, and Thai establishments. Olive oil, along with lemon and some balsamic vinegar, is probably the best salad dressing you can use when eating out. Always order it, as well as sauces, on the side. Use just 1 tablespoon. You can drizzle a little bit on your entrée as well as on your salad.

Seafoods, as you know by now, are a great source of omega-3 fatty acids. You may select from a wide variety of fish and seafood. Of course, salmon (both the Atlantic and king varieties) is the "king" of the omega-3s. You can get salmon fresh pretty much anywhere these days. Other high-omega-3 fish you can try include mackerel, rainbow trout, halibut, cod, haddock, tuna, and believe it or not, anchovies. Although a bit salty, the lowly anchovy is high in omega-3 fat-burning power. Salmon and other fish can be grilled, broiled, poached, or baked in wine and seasoned with lots of fresh garlic (specify fresh; otherwise, garlic salt will be used) and onions. Some Japanese and Chinese dishes use peanut oil for stir-frying. This is also acceptable. A delicious Fat Flush smart choice in Mexican restaurants is guacamole, which contains beneficial monounsaturated fats similar to those in olive oil. It can be used as a topping, in place of sour cream or heavy cheese. Just remember to "lemonize" whenever and wherever you can, which I believe cuts the fat and assists in metabolism.

The Entrée

In addition to the omega-3 fish, seafood, poultry, beef, lamb, and veal, you also can have a tempeh or tofu dish a couple of times a week. These are always best either grilled or steamed.

You may want to accompany your entrée with a salad, but hold those croutons. They are usually made with hydrogenated oil just like the prepared salad dressings. A double portion of steamed veggies (preferably fresh) and a friendly carb for those on phase 2 or Lifestyle Fat Flush (such as cooked carrots, peas, a small baked potato, brown rice, or corn on the cob with a small amount of your flaxseed oil blended with the real butter at the table) are good choices. And be sure to ask if that's really butter on the table—not an imitation. Ration yourself to one pat. Side orders of roasted garlic, parsley, chives, leeks, and even chopped onions can be an added flavor booster for your meal.

For breakfast, eggs that are poached or boiled (hard or soft) are a good choice. Or have them prepared as an omelet with lots of fresh veggies such as onions, spinach, and peppers. Although not ideal because of the high sodium and additive content in some of these selections, other breakfast foods that will work on the road are lox or smoked salmon, turkey sausage, cottage cheese, and a couple of slices of real Swiss cheese with tomatoes. If you're hankering for a whole-grain cereal but aren't on the Lifestyle Fat Flush Plan yet, make sure you have enough protein and fat (such as a scoop of cottage cheese) to provide a balance so that you don't overdo the crash-and-burn carbohydrates. Otherwise, you'll wind up looking for a pick-me-up an hour later from sugar or a caffeine-laden beverage such as coffee, tea, or cola.

And speaking of caffeine and beverages, here's the lowdown. Although I know that green tea has been touted as a miracle drink, high in the phenol-based antioxidants that help to prevent certain types of cancer, my feeling is that caffeine is caffeine is caffeine—a theme reiterated throughout this book! There are 35 mg of caffeine in 6 ounces of green tea versus 100 mg in a 6-ounce cup of drip-brewed coffee. Besides, most teas are high in copper, the mineral that seems to go hand in hand with estrogen, resulting in estrogen excess and water retention.

If you are in the Lifestyle Fat Flush phase, I would suggest selecting or bringing your own herbal tea bags, such as peppermint or hibiscus tea. You also could bring along dandelion or red tea (rooibos tea), an antioxidant-rich tea that is also good for balancing blood sugar levels. Red tea comes from South Africa, where it has been enjoyed for over 200 years. It is high in the antioxidant-rich flavonoids. In fact, both it and dandelion tea nourish your liver.

The second-best option might be a blended herbal green tea, which cuts down on the caffeine because it also contains herbs. I would look for Tazo Om and Green Ginger, The Republic of Tea Moroccan Mint, or Celestial Seasonings Green Tea with Antioxidants.

Avoid iced teas or iced-tea mixes, because they are often presweetened with lots of sugar or aspartame. A much simpler alternative is to order hot water with lemon or lime. Just remember: When in doubt, "lemonize"! There is something fresh and clean about lemons and limes. I think you'll agree with me that they are quite satisfying.

FAT FLUSHING IN THE FAST-FOOD LANE

As far as take-out meals are concerned, there are some okay meals that don't exactly conform to the Fat Flushing principles but are acceptable in a pinch—once you're on the Lifestyle Fat Flush eating phase, that is. Some examples are the grilled chicken sandwiches at Arby's, Dairy Queen, Hardee's, or Carl's (9 g of fat, 28 g of protein, and 33 g of carbohydrate); the chicken fajita pita at Jack-in-the-Box (9 g of fat, 28 g of protein, and 31 g of carbohydrate); and the chili at Wendy's (8 g of fat, 24 g of protein, and 29 g of carbohydrate). Of course, try your best to eat your fast-food sandwiches open face and avoid eating the bread and eat only half of the pita, even if you are in the Lifestyle phase. Both the bread and the pita are most likely made from white flour, and empty calorie eating is a Fat Flush no-no.

And, as mentioned previously, no matter what phase of the plan you are on, I would definitely look for places that feature rotisserie chicken or turkey, touted as a much healthier alternative to the fried version because the fat drips off when the meat is on a rotating spit. With a side salad and steamed vegetables plus lots of fresh lemon, you can't beat it.

You also should be on the lookout for Rubios (www.rubios.com), a chain spreading all over the country, which is the home of the fish taco. The grilled fish is made from mahi mahi or red snapper and comes in a delightful yogurt-type sauce with fresh cabbage. Ask for a corn tortilla instead of the taco shell. In Lifestyle a corn tortilla counts as 1 friendly carb, but taco shells are loaded with trans fats. I usually order several fish tacos and remove the taco shells. Rubios also has lots of salsas and fresh lime for seasonings.

Most of the other fast-food items I have evaluated are way too high in saturated fats, which you want to keep in balance. Bacon, for example, and regular salad dressings are 75 percent fat; cheesecake is 70 percent fat. A taco salad (with the shell) is 60 percent fat, as are fried shrimp, fried chicken wings and thighs, a bacon cheeseburger, and an egg-and-meat croissant. Again, Boston Market and other establishments that feature rotisserie chicken and turkey are some of the better fast-food choices. Of course, you can always visit a Wendy's and prepare a salad from the salad bar and/or order a grilled chicken sandwich or hamburger with lettuce, onions, and mustard. Just remember to remove the bun!

Speak Up

Don't be shy. Make your personal needs known to your server in a nice way. Ask a question such as "Do you serve butter or margarine?" or "What are the ingredients in this dish?" And always ask for the butter, olive oil, and sauces on the side.

Also ask about methods used to prepare foods, and make it quite clear that you don't want anything that is fried (a sure bet for getting those nasty trans fats). You may want to find out what kind of fresh vegetables are available and request that they be steamed. I always look on the menu and find what veggies are served with other dishes and then politely ask if they can be included with my entrée too. This approach has been especially important for me when I can't get greens readily. For instance, I search for a dish that has sautéed spinach or escarole with garlic and then make my request.

Let your server know that you definitely don't want margarine added to your broiled or grilled entrées, which is frequently done to avoid dryness. Ditto for mayonnaise, which also is likely to have the trans fats. You can add a pat of butter if you are on the Lifestyle phase.

GOING ETHNIC

You can enjoy Italian, Chinese, Mexican, French, Japanese, Middle Eastern, Indian, and Thai cuisine on the Fat Flush Plan. Cajun and Creole foods are not off limits either for special occasions. Just keep in mind that highly spicy foods can cause water retention in some people.

Italian

This is the cuisine where you have to watch overdoing carbs such as pasta, beans, and that delicious garlic bread. Thus, you might want to have the server take the bread basket away as soon as you sit down. If you are really hungry, then order an appetizer right away. Grilled portobello mushrooms or an artichoke (hold the breading) is a tasty starter. You may want to indulge in a Caesar salad, which is perfectly Fat Flush legal. Just ask for it without croutons and get the dressing on the side. And if you have a taste for anchovies, go for it! They are high in the omega-3s, although a bit on the salty side. The best news at an Italian restaurant is that you usually can get a wide variety of delicious, colorful veggies that are not as easily available elsewhere, such as zucchini, peppers, cauliflower, eggplant, and spaghetti squash. In addition, typically you can get a leafy green, such as spinach or escarole, here as well. Sautéed with onions, fresh garlic, and a little lemon in olive oil or chicken broth, these vegetables are out of this world and very Fat Flush friendly.

And oh yes, there's that cheese—the mozzarella, ricotta, and provolone. For those of you on the Lifestyle Fat Flush eating plan, keep them to a tasty minimum and use them as a condiment, please. You can even have your pesto (that sensational combination of olive oil, garlic, basil, pine nuts, and Parmesan cheese) and eat it too. Ask for it on the side so that you can enjoy a couple of tablespoons slowly and deliberately. Do not overlook the veal dishes (the Marsala, piccata, or scaloppini), which are usually quite outstanding in the finer Italian restaurants. Since Italian dishes can be on the oily side, learn to "lemonize" by ordering several lemon wedges that can help emulsify excess oil.

Chinese

Things are really simple when you go Chinese. Just find out which dishes can be made to order, and request no monosodium glutamate (MSG), sugar, salt, or soy sauce. If you must, you can always add your own soy sauce at the table. If the oil is anything other than sesame or peanut oil, then order your food steamed. I always request a stir-fry using chicken broth made from such combinations as beef, chicken, seafood, or tofu with snow peas, water chestnuts, bean sprouts, broccoli, scallions, bamboo shoots, and bok choy (Chinese cabbage.)

If you are in the Lifestyle phase and want a good vegetarian meal, try Buddha's Delight, a mix of vegetables and rice cellophane noodles which can be stir-sautéed in vegetable broth. Buddha's Delight can be modified for any Fat Flush phase by omitting the noodles. You can have tofu added to the dish with a side of steamed veggies topped off with scallions, garlic, and a bit of Chinese Five Spice powder, a delightful mixture of exotic spices related to cinnamon. Most of the soups offered in a Chinese restaurant are made with lots of cornstarch—including egg drop soup—so it is best to skip the soup course. On the Lifestyle Fat Flush, lo mein dishes, the cellophane or mung bean noodles with some chicken, beef, shrimp, or other kinds of seafood, also might be appealing. Just remember that those oyster and black bean sauces are loaded with salt, which can result in boggy, watery tissues. Try a bit of the hot mustard, minced garlic, scallions, and even some Chinese Five Spice powder instead.

As for the fortune cookie—by all means have fun and open it. Read your fortune, and then leave the cookie behind. Also, try eating with chopsticks. It may help to slow you down and enhance your digestion as a result.

Mexican

You may want to select such entrées as chicken, shrimp, or beef and eat them without the tortilla unless you are on the Lifestyle Fat Flush. Look for main dishes with fish, chicken, or beef that can be prepared with onions, tomatoes, and peppers (such as Veracruz snapper) or those which can be sautéed in olive oil with a touch of garlic. If you are on the Lifestyle

Fat Flush, a tasty Mexican soup (such as black bean soup) would be a great way to start your meal. If not, then how about some guacamole (loaded with the healthy monounsaturated fats) with lots of fresh lemon or lime juice? Salsa is probably your best all-over topping. Use the sour cream and cheese as condiments, with just a dollop or a few sprinkles here and there for flavor. If you are fortunate enough to locate an authentic Mexican restaurant, such foods as squash blossoms, jícama, and chayote cactus are treats for the palate.

French

Oo-la-la! Here you can select from a wide variety of broiled, poached, and steamed foods. Anything sautéed in a wine sauce, such as a Bordelaise sauce, is bound to be a winner. The traditional French dish fish en papillote (cooked with herbs in its own juices) is highly recommended, as are such dishes as roast chicken with herbs (poulet aux fines herbes), ratatouille (a vegetable casserole), bouillabaisse, and coq au vin. Poached salmon is also a tasty choice, but go light on the butter and cream sauce in this and other selections. Try to stay away from dishes featuring duck. They are usually quite fatty and laden with sauces that are quite sweet.

Japanese

As in Chinese cuisine, these dishes tend to feature soy sauce, which should be avoided as much as possible because of its high salt content. For the same reason, you will need to go light on the teriyaki sauce (a blend of soy sauce, rice wine, and sugar) and sukiyaki, which are used as marinades for many entrées featuring chicken and beef. Similarly, miso (the fermented soybean paste) is also high in salt. A bit of miso, however, can be used as a glaze or as a soup base with sea vegetables (hijiki and arame) and scallions.

Japanese restaurants are known for their sushi bars. Choose your sushi or sashimi, with care because raw fish often can be contaminated with parasites. (Please refer to my book, *Guess What Came to Dinner.*) Lifestylers can go for the California rolls (avocado and cooked shrimp) and for that matter can also enjoy any sushi offerings that are made with smoked salmon or cooked crab, cooked shrimp, cooked egg, cooked eel, and cooked octopus. Straight vegetarian sushi (such as the kappa maki, made with cucumbers) is good too. The nori seaweed wrapping surrounding all these delights is quite nutritious in its own right—and it's loaded with trace minerals. Of course, if brown rice is used in the sushi—all the better.

The best strategy for eating Japanese cuisine is going for the grilled entrées of scallops, shrimp, chicken, and beef, which are prepared using the hibachi grill. Hibachi-style food preparation has become quite popular.

I believe that the popular restaurateur Benihana pioneered this method with his line of Japanese restaurants. Now there are Mongolian-style barbecue outlets popping up all over the country featuring this method of cooking. You can build your own meal from a variety of fresh ingredients (e.g., raw beef, chicken, shrimp, and scallops) with lots of vegetables and even sesame seeds, however you like it. As long as there is plenty of fresh garlic, parsley, and scallions, you really can't go wrong.

Mediterranean/Greek

Pita (pocket) bread is served routinely in these restaurants along with two savory vegetarian dips, hummus and babaghanoush. Hummus is a chickpea paté; babaghanoush is eggplant paté. Both are made with sesame butter, garlic, and lemon. Blended with some tzatziki (yogurt and cucumbers), each can serve as a salad dressing, or just the tzatziki alone will do the honors. I would skip the pita entirely, because it is usually made from refined white flour, which as you well know is not recommended on any phase of the Fat Flush Plan. Instead, use celery sticks and cucumbers for the dips.

If you're on the Lifestyle Fat Flush and are not wheat intolerant, you also might enjoy a flavorful grain salad known as *tabouleh*, made with bulgur wheat, parsley, onion, tomatoes, olive oil, lemon, and mint. Greek salads and others that feature feta (goat) cheese are also a nutritious choice. Try a spinach pie for a satisfying taste treat. As a great main course for all Fat Flushers, try shish kabob (grilled meat and vegetables). Or if you like it hot, souvlakis (skewered lamb, beef, chicken, and fish kabobs) are the ticket. Sides of chopped parsley, tomatoes, and scallions with mint and lots of lemon can top off a lovely meal.

Indian

Indian cuisine featuring pilafs and biryanis (rice-based dishes) and bean-based dals is okay in moderation if you're on the Lifestyle Fat Flush, of course. Tandoori chicken and lamb, which are cooked in a clay oven to retain the moisture from the meat, are also fine for phases 1 and 2. Other tasty entrées for Lifestylers include chicken or lamb korma with coriander and yogurt sauce. Lightly curried vegetable and chicken dishes will satisfy those who like spicy foods and do not retain water from hot seasoning.

The Indian dal salad is similar to tabouleh, but is made with lentils instead of wheat. Remember that the lentils are friendly carbs—so figure them into your meals regularly. Or you can enjoy instead a couple (and only a couple) of baked pappadums (lentil wafers). The chapati and nan (garlic and onion breads) are very delicious but are also made from wheat, so it is best to stay away from them entirely if you know that you are sensitive to wheat.

Thai

This is a personal favorite. You can basically follow the recommendations outlined above for Indian cuisine, but you may wish to add the popular coconut milk–based soups such as tom kha. Enjoy it with some protein, such as shrimp, chicken, or beef. Coconut actually contains a healthful, naturally saturated fat known for its antiviral properties. You can enjoy these soups with lemongrass and cilantro seasonings when you are on Lifestyle.

In closing, after eating the Fat Flush way for years, I can say that the best way to eat out is to ask questions and even shop around for a restaurant that is responsive to your special requests. In Santa Fe, a Chinese restaurant used to keep a special bottle of sesame oil and cook all dishes in this oil for my family and guests. In San Diego, one of the Chinese restaurants added brown rice to the menu. The owners were more than happy to comply with my special requests, especially when I brought in huge parties of friends and publicly thanked them again for making my life so much healthier.

PARTIES, BUSINESS LUNCHEONS, AND HOLIDAY EVENTS

The holiday season? No problem, especially on Lifestyle. You just need to know the inside tips. For starters, eat a little something before you arrive. In this way, you won't be famished and tempted to eat the sugary, starchy pick-me-ups or appetizers that undoubtedly will surround you. Grab a glass of mineral water and hold it in your hand—getting refills as needed—throughout the evening. No one will notice you're not drinking alcohol. And, of course, for those really festive times, indulge in some spirits. Light beer—maybe 6 ounces or so—an ounce of hard liquor, and even a half glassful of dry wine are allowable. Just don't drink on an empty stomach. Have your drinks with some vegetables and dip, with cheese, or with dinner.

Business luncheons can be a snap. First, there's usually a salad. The safest dressings are the vinaigrettes. Remember to always order them on the side. You never know about the blue cheese and ranch dressings, which may be made with trans-fat mayonnaise. You can always squeeze fresh lemon on your salad whenever in doubt. I personally order a Caesar salad because I am assured that the lettuce is really green. Romaine is higher in nutrients such as heart-healthy and bone-healthy magnesium and chlorophyll than its lack-luster relatives, particularly iceberg.

If you can manage it, just ask for a double helping of the vegetables with your entrée in place of the white rice, pasta, or baked potato you can pretty much bet will be part of your meal. Remember these are the carbs that can raise your blood sugar levels quickly, especially if there's not enough protein or healthy fat to balance the surge.

If fresh fruit is for dessert (fresh berries to be exact), you're home free. I always ask for fresh berries even if they are not on the menu. Most of the time they are available, especially in finer establishments.

The important thing here is not to make a big deal about your food preferences and draw attention to yourself. If you do, anyone else who knows better but isn't following healthy principles will redirect their guilt and make you feel uncomfortable. It will be evident in their looks and facial expressions. I know; I have been there many times.

If a buffet is on the menu, then go out of your way to avoid the potato, pasta, and three-bean salads (which often have some added sugar to boot). Then run to the protein. Freshly carved roast beef, grilled or baked fish, chicken dishes, lamb, and the like should be your basic favorites. Check out the veggie section, choosing any green veggie you want to fill up your plate: spinach, broccoli, asparagus, and green beans. If you are a phase 2 or are a Lifestyle Fat Flush eater, then select one friendly carb (and only one) to accompany your meal based on the Fat Flushing friendly carb choices.

The holidays may feel like a minefield of problems, but they don't have to be. You actually can join in the festivities, eat smart, *and* keep that Fat Flush shape. I know that traditionally during those special times of the year—particularly from Thanksgiving and Christmas to New Year's—many of us have let down our guard and packed on 10 to 15 pounds. Here are some ways to sidestep those holiday pounds and still have fun celebrating with your family and friends.

The first thing you'll want to do is continue taking your conjugated linoleic acid (CLA), because even with a slipup, half the weight you regain will be redeposited as muscle. Then, about an hour before you hit the holiday scene, have a salad or, if you are on Lifestyle, a bowl of soup to curb your appetite. You might want to try circulating around the room and meeting new people. Not only will it be interesting and fun, but it also will keep you from hanging out near the food. While you're making the rounds at a party, scan the food table and look for smart Fat Flush food choices. When you want to nibble on something, select raw veggies rather than the carb-rich crackers and trans-fatty chips. It's also a good idea to use a napkin, not a plate, so that you eat less. And while you're there, head on over to that dance floor and get groovin'! Dancing is great exercise and a real calorie burner.

On Lifestyle, at work, where everyone seems to bring in all kinds of goodies during the holiday season, bypass the cookies and candy. Select a handful of raw nuts and fruit instead. If you are having the holiday meal at your home or if you are bringing a dish to someone else's home, cook up some mashed sweet potatoes seasoned with cinnamon instead of those candied yams. Make a Fat Flush dip, serving it with celery, cucumber, and zucchini sticks. Forget the bread stuffing and use a variety of seeds, nuts, and vegetables (such as celery, onions, and mushrooms seasoned with anise, cayenne, garlic, or parsley).

And since the holidays are an especially stressful time of year—stirring up one of those hidden weight gain factors that piles on the pounds—be sure to keep your diet nutrient-dense so that blood sugar levels remain steady. Keep a keen eye out for hidden sugars, and be sure to consume adequate protein and fat to balance your body's chemistry.

I also recommend getting the helpful yeast-fighter Y-C Cleanse. It will help keep cravings at an all-time low. (See Chapter 12.) This is extremely important because all those holiday cakes, cookies, and candies contain sugar, which is the favorite food of yeast. By keeping your yeast in check, you will lose your appetite for such goodies. For years I have recommended Y-C Cleanse as a preventive measure against holiday weight gain. And it really works.

Enjoy!

CHAPTER

9 The Master Fat Flush Shopping List

We've added so many preservatives, nutrients, artificial coloring, and chemicals that there's no room for the product.

—CHICAGO TRIBUNE

Fat Flush really begins when you start to clean up and clear out your kitchen. The goal is to replace old habits with new ones. The first step is to replace old, familiar products with newer, better ones.

To help you get started on your Fat Flush journey, here's the complete Fat Flush Plan shopping list with brand names for the tastiest and most convenient Fat Flush foods currently available. This all-in-one shopping list contains the foods you can eat in all three phases of the program, which, are noted as such. The first several pages contain the approved products for phase 1 (the Two-Week Fat Flush). Next, you will see the products you can add for phase 2, the Ongoing Fat Flush. The final section includes all the additional products appropriate for phase 3, the Lifestyle Eating Plan.

Keep in mind that many of these foods can be purchased at your local health food store, whereas others are available in supermarkets. The omega-3–enriched eggs listed are definitely worth the modest price increase, not to mention the superior, rich, and creamy taste of the brightly colored yolk. Naturally, organic produce (vegetables and fruit) are preferred when possible (not only are they tastier and fresher, but they do not have all those nasty pesticides, fungicides, and heavy metals your liver has to break down). For this reason, I am providing the names of some of the easier-to-obtain brands in parentheses. And of course, if you have access to conjugated linoleic acid (CLA)–rich meats and dairy products, then opt for grass-fed beef, poultry, and lamb as much as possible to maximize your body's fat loss. You will find a listing by state of all the suppliers of grass-fed meat in Chapter 12.

Now, if organic foods are not within your budget or not available in your locale, don't despair. I will share with you the names of some veggie washes you can purchase at your local grocery store or health food store. Also, at the end of this chapter you'll find a tried-and-true food-cleansing bath designed to return farm freshness to store-bought food.

Items that are readily available throughout the country in either health food stores or supermarkets are listed simply by brand name. Others that are not as readily available have a telephone number and Web site added for you to get further information.

You will also find information about the herbal coffees mentioned in Chapter 3. I have included a more comprehensive listing in the protein section than is found in the preceding chapters to help you vary your menu planning and select the best cuts of meat. You will find a specific listing of the veggie and fruit options in the sections entitled "Phase 1," "Phase 2," and "Phase 3." Now let's get shopping!

BEFORE YOU BEGIN

Herbal Coffee Substitute: Naturally caffeine-free herbal coffee blended from herbs, grains, fruits, and nuts. Available from Teeccino at 1-800-498-3434, or visit www.teeccino.com.

INSIDER TIP

Teeccino is brewed like regular coffee and comes in seven flavors, Java, Original, Hazelnut, Vanilla Nut, Amaretto, Mocha, and Chocolate Mint. The lowest carb flavors are Java, Vanilla Nut, and Hazelnut at 3 g of carb per serving and Mocha at 4 g.

During the first couple of days, I felt sluggish. But by day 10, I had more energy and felt better than I had in a long time. And in just fourteen days, I dropped 19 pounds, then an additional 5 pounds by maintaining Fat Flush principles, the cranberry-water drink, and supplements. That totaled 24 pounds and 6 inches—and I went from a size 16 to a 10!

I also noticed I wasn't waking up several times during the night, the way I used to before going on Fat Flush. My clothes fit great, and I am feeling pretty terrific. Now I stick to eating the way Fat Flush taught me, choosing salmon, tuna, chicken, and lots of salads. And I have lost my desire for those carbonated beverages I used to crave. I even joined a women's fitness group!

—Reba Caraway

PHASE 1: THE TWO-WEEK FAT FLUSH

Oil: High-lignan flaxseed oil. Fat Flushers seem to prefer Omega Nutrition, Spectrum, Flora, and Health from the Sun.

STORAGE TIP | Keep in fridge. An 8-ounce bottle lasts for about three weeks.

Eggs: Omega-3–enriched. (Gold Circle Farms, The Country Hen, Eggland's Best, Born 3, Pilgrim's Pride EggsPlus).

HEALTH TIP | These incredible eggs contain twenty times more omega-3s than their supermarket sisters. Both The Country Hen and Pilgrim's Pride EggsPlus contain about 200 mg of this essential fatty acid.

Protein powders: Lactose-free, no-sugar-added 100 percent whey protein (Naturade 100% Whey Protein, Solgar's Whey to Go, Designer Whey Protein, American Sports Nutrition American Whey).

Lean-protein fish: All fresh, especially bass, cod, grouper, haddock, halibut, mackerel, mahi mahi, orange roughy, perch, pike, pollock, salmon, sardines, sole, snapper, trout, tuna, and whitefish, and canned tuna, salmon, mackerel, sardines, and crabmeat (Featherweight, Seasons, Lillie, Three Star).

HEALTH TIP | If packed in oil or with added salt, drain well under running water.

Seafood: Shrimp, lobster, crab, scallops, calamari.

HEALTH TIP | If shrimp or crab is canned, then drain well under running water to remove excess salt.

Poultry: White meat of skinned turkey and chicken, either fresh, frozen, or ground (preferably free-range and hormone-free, such as Foster Farms, Harmony Farms, Shelton Farms, and Young Farms; also see Chapter 12).

Beef: Flank, rump, round, eye of the round, chuck, brisket, sirloin, and London broil. (Belle Brooke Farms in Nacogdoches, Texas, at 1-409-560-9482 has the most delicious beef I have ever tasted. Their beef is "certified" and fed without antibiotics, growth stimulants, or animal by-products.)

Lamb: Leg, loin, rib.

Veal: Shoulder, rib, loin.

Other meats: Venison, ostrich, bison (or buffalo), and elk.

HEALTH TIP | **These meats can be substituted for the protein in any recipe and are higher in the fat-burning omega-3s than their commercial counterparts.**

Other protein sources: Tempeh and tofu (Mori-Nu and White Wave).

Vegetables: All fresh, in-season produce that is green, red, orange, or purple. (Fresh is always best, followed by frozen and then canned with no added salt. Bamboo shoots, water chestnuts, and artichoke hearts are Fat Flush friendly either canned or frozen. Frozen brands are Cascadian Farms and Stahlbush Island Farms.)

Fruits: Fresh (without mold), frozen, or canned in natural unsweetened juices and drained (frozen brands include Cascadian Farms and Stahlbush Island Farms).

Lemons: Fresh is best, although Santa Cruz Organic 100% Lemon Juice Not From Concentrate will do.

Limes: Fresh is best, although Santa Cruz Organic 100% Lime Juice Not From Concentrate will do.

HEALTH TIP | **One tablespoon equals the juice of one-half lemon or lime.**

Cooking broths: Low-sodium or no-salt-added beef, chicken, fish, or vegetable broths (Shelton's, Health Valley, Hain's, and Perfect Addition).

HEALTH TIP

Shelton's low-sodium chicken broth contains 60 mg of sodium per cup, whereas Health Valley's no-salt-added chicken broth contains nearly twice this amount at 130 mg per cup. Hain's no-salt-added chicken broth has 140 mg per cup. Health Valley's no-salt-added beef broth contains 120 mg per cup. A frozen line of unsalted beef, chicken, fish, and vegetable stock concentrates is now available in health food stores in the frozen foods section.

Perfect Addition, from Newport Beach, California, is a Fat Flusher's dream, with the only unsalted vegetable concentrate I could find without monosodium glutamate (MSG), which is a neurotoxin. MSG is also found in such products as texturized vegetable protein, gelatin, maltodextrin, yeast extract, yeast food, and autolyzed yeast.

Herbs, spices, and accompaniments: Apple cider vinegar, cayenne, cinnamon, cloves, coriander (dried cilantro) cumin, dill, dried mustard, garlic, ginger, fennel, anise, bay leaves, and fresh jalapenos (optional), as well as Dave's Gourmet Roasted Garlic and Eggplant Spread. (It's exquisite for dipping veggies. I love it on eggs! Call 1-800-758-0372.)

Tomato products: Muir Glen Tomato Puree, Muir Glen No Salt Added Diced Tomatoes, Muir Glen No Salt Added Tomato Sauce, Muir Glen Tomato Paste, Muir Glen Whole Peeled Tomatoes, and Muir Glen Pizza Sauce. (Check out a complete list of Muir Glen Organic Products at *www.muirglen.com*.)

HEALTH TIP

Millina's Healthy Kitchen Marinara, Tomato Garlic, and Tomato Basil are enriched with omega-3s (call 1-866-492-5688).

Long Life Cocktail: Powdered psyllium husks (Yerba Prima or other health food bulk brands) or ground flaxseeds (Nutri Flax and Certified Organic Milled Flaxseeds).

Flaxseeds: Whole brown or golden yellow flaxseeds in bulk to be ground daily as needed in a coffee grinder, blender, or food processor on the fine setting.

Cranberry juice: Unsweetened cranberry juice (Knudsen's, Trader Joe's, Mountain Sun).

Sweeteners: Herbal sweeteners (Stevia Plus). (Stevia Plus comes in a shaker bottle and packets, perfect when you're going out to eat. Call 1-800-899-9908, or visit the company's Web site at *www.steviaplus.com*.)

HEALTH TIP

Stevia Plus is the only natural sweetener (including all other Stevia offerings I have tasted) with no "funky" aftertaste. In addition, Stevia Plus does not contain maltodextrin, a high-glycemic-index sugar, like other Stevia offerings. The addition of the friendly bacteria–nourishing fructooligosaccharides (FOSs) adds even more fiber without more bulk.

Water: Purified, ozonated, and/or electrolyte (magnesium and potassium) enhanced water. (Trinity, Essentia, Aquafina, Dani, or water from a home filtration system; Trinity is the only certified spring water in the United States which also meets European standards.)

PHASE 2: ONGOING FAT FLUSH

You may have these foods in addition to the ones on the phase 1 list.

Sprouted breads: Wheat-free, yeast-free bread with sprouted grains and legumes (HealthSeed Spelt from French Meadow Bakery, Ezekiel 4:9 from Rainier and Food for Life, and Sprouted Multigrain from Alvarado Street Bakery).

HEALTH TIP

HealthSeed Spelt is packed with flax, pumpkin, and sunflower seeds for added crunch. Instead of yeast, the bread is naturally leavened with fermenting agents that break down the flour's cellulose structure, neutralize its mineral-inhibiting phytic acid, and release more nutrients into the dough. HealthSeed Spelt contains 18 g of carbohydrate (13 g after 5 g of fiber are deducted). The Ezekiel 4:9 sprouted-grain bread is also a flourless whole-grain bread that I have recommended for years. It does have a small amount of sweeteners (either molasses or malted barley). One slice of Ezekiel 4:9 sprouted-grain bread contains 14 g of carbohydrate (11 g after the fiber grams are deducted). One slice of Alvarado Street Bakery's Sprouted Multigrain Bread contains only 11 g of carbohydrate (9 g after the fiber grams are deducted). It is made from organically grown sprouted wheat berries; filtered water; an organically grown grain mixture consisting of millet, rye flakes, cornmeal, rolled oats, and barley flakes; pure honey; unsulfured molasses; lecithin; wheat gluten; and fresh yeast.

Friendly carbs: Sweet potato, frozen or fresh peas, carrots, and butternut and acorn squash.

I'm a thirty-eight-year-old man. My wife found your diet program, and after seeing her results the first week, I decided to give it a try myself. I have lost almost all the extra fat around my midsection. I look and feel like I'm eighteen again!

I did modify the diet slightly, added more protein, and increased the portions slightly. I just wanted to tell you how thankful I am that I discovered your program. Thanks!

—Craig in California

PHASE 3: LIFESTYLE EATING PLAN

You may have these foods in addition to the ones on the phase 1 and 2 lists.

Lean protein: Frozen fish burgers (Northwest Naturals).

HEALTH TIP Northwest Natural produces three kinds of frozen fish medallions—salmon, halibut, and tuna with pesto—all of which are omega-3 sources. The wild rice in these medallions makes these burgers suitable for the Lifestyle Eating Plan.

Beef: Beef jerky (Shelton's).

Turkey: Turkey jerky (Shelton's).

HEALTH TIP Shelton's beef and turkey jerky are without MSG, nitrates, or corn sugar and are nicely processed in a tamari-based blend.

Nuts and seeds: Raw almonds, filberts, pecans, peanuts, walnuts, macadamia nuts, pumpkin seeds (Pumpkorn at 1-800-431-4018 or *www.pumpkorn.com*), sunflower seeds, poppy seeds, and caraway, as well as peanut, almond, and sesame butters or tahina (Arrowhead Mills, Westbrae).

STORAGE TIP Store nuts and seeds in a cool, dry place such as the fridge or freezer. Home-toast all seeds and nuts in the oven for fifteen minutes at 250°F to help set the oil.

Mayonnaise: Spectrum Naturals organic mayonnaise.

Dairy products: Nonfat or plain yogurt, cottage cheese (Friendship, Old Home), ricotta cheese (Calabro), Swiss, Cheddar, grated Parmesan (occasionally), string cheese, mozzarella, goat cheese, sweet butter, and cream.

HEALTH TIP Companies such as Nancy's and Horizon offer a wide variety of organic dairy products.

Friendly carbs: Corn tortillas, corn chips, corn on the cob, potatoes, chickpeas, pinto beans, black beans, kidney beans, brown rice, whole-grain pasta, popcorn.

Crackers: Scandinavian-style crisp breads without trans fats (Bran-A-Crisp, Kavli, and Wasa).

> **HEALTH TIP** Bran-A-Crisp and Kavli crackers contain 4 g of carbohydrate per cracker, and Wasa light rye crackers have 5 g of carbohydrate per cracker.

Vegetable juice: Low-sodium vegetable juices (Low Sodium V-8 Juice, Muir Glen Tomato Juice, Muir Glen 100% Vegetable Juice, and Knudsen Organic Very Veggie Juice).

Flavor extracts: Sugarless vanilla and chocolate extracts [Nielsen-Massey Sugarless Vanilla Extract, Lochhead Vanilla (314-772-2124), and Star Kay White's Pure Chocolate Extract (*www.atkinscenter.com*)].

> **HEALTH TIP** Chock full of the essence of cocoa beans without the sugar and without the fat.

Salt: Mineral-enhanced or sea salt (Cardia Salt, Celtic Salt, Real Salt, Bioforce Herbamare Salt, and Trocomare Herbal Salt).

> **INSIDER TIP** I really prefer Cardia Salt, which has less than half the sodium of table salt with potassium and magnesium and actually tastes just like salt! Use measure for measure, just like salt (call 1-888-422-7342).

Herbs, spices, and condiments: Oregano, basil, sage, savory, rosemary, tarragon, thyme, Chinese Five Spice powder, Dijon mustard, Angostura bitters, and capers.

Acceptable teas and coffees: Dandelion root and red tea (rooibos tea), organic coffee (Allegro Organic Coffee and Allegro Organic Decaf [1-800-277-1107]), decaffeinated green tea, rosehip tea, fennel tea, taheebo (good for yeast control), peppermint tea, and hibiscus tea (Tazo Om and Green Ginger, The Republic of Tea Moroccan Mint, Celestial Seasonings Green Tea with Antioxidants).

Alcohol: Organic and sulfite-free (Frey, Fetzer, Summerhill Estate Winery, Organic Wine Company, HoneyRun Winery, Hallcrest Vineyards, and Chinabend Vineyards, available at health food stores and gourmet outlets).

HEALTH TIP For that special occasion and cooking. When these wines are used as cooking wines, the flavor remains and the alcohol evaporates.

Oils and sprays: Extra virgin and unfiltered olive oils (Kroger, Bertolli, Private Selection, Oligra, Mezzetta, and Sasso), sesame and toasted sesame oils (Spectrum and Eden), rice bran oil (Tsuno), and olive oil sprays.

STORAGE TIP Both olive and sesame oils can be kept in a cool, dark place.

Baking powder: Aluminum-free brands (Royal, Rumford, Price, and Schillings) and low-sodium, cereal-free brands (Cellu and Featherweight).

Thickeners: Arrowroot and kudzu (available in bulk at health food stores).

FOOD-CLEANSING BATHS

If organic foods are unavailable or simply too expensive, there are many new fruit and vegetable cleansers on the market that can be found in grocery and health food stores. One such cleanser is Bi-O-Kleen, containing grapefruit seed extract that kills bacteria such as *Escherichia coli.* Bi-O-Kleen can be reached at 1-503-557-0216 or *www.bi-o-kleen.com.* Another alternative is Organiclean. This company can be reached by calling 1-888-834-9274 or going to *www.organiclean.com.*

Dr. Parcells' Food Bath

There is, however, another alternative you may be interested in trying. It's called a *Clorox bath* (yes, as in Clorox bleach). It is a definite option for produce as well as poultry, fish, meat, and eggs. As many of my faithful readers know, since the introduction of the Clorox bath back in my first book, *Beyond Pritikin,* in 1988, based on Dr. Parcells' research, pesticides, parasites, bacteria (such as *Salmonella*), and other contaminants can be removed from food with this simple soak. Please note that Clorox is not the same as chlorine, the chemical disinfectant added to drinking water, which has been linked to heart disease and cancer. In fact, the active ingredient in Clorox, sodium hypochlorite, breaks down into salt and water.

Dr. Parcells discovered the oxygenating value of the Clorox bath while she was the head of the Nutrition Department at the Sierra State University (a naturopathic college at the time) back in the 1960s. The story goes that a friend brought her a bunch of shriveled lemons, which she decided to dump in water with some Clorox for some unknown reason. Amazingly, within a half hour, the lemons regenerated and plumped up. Dr. Parcells surmised that the Clorox enabled the lemons to take in oxygen and become fresh once again.

The Clorox bath has been around for decades, and military families stationed overseas in Southeast Asia, China, and Turkey have used it through the recommendation of our State Department.

Over the years, my readers and clients who have used this method report that foods last up to two weeks longer in the refrigerator, there is no metallic aftertaste with store-bought fruits and veggies, and meats are tenderized and their natural flavors enhanced.

Here is the Clorox cleansing bath that Dr. Parcells recommended, which I continue to use in my own home. To ensure quality, I use only brand-name Clorox, since Dr. Parcells was very clear that other brands were not effective. For those of you who are familiar with the bath and remember the formula to contain ½ teaspoon of Clorox to 1 gallon of water, Dr. Parcells increased the Clorox amount to 1 teaspoon shortly before her death in 1996. She said the increasing chemicals and bacteria in our foods made it necessary to double the Clorox.

The formula: Use 1 teaspoon of Clorox to 1 gallon of purified, ozonated, and/or electrolyte-enhanced water. Place the foods to be treated into the bath for the designated length of time according to the following chart. Remove the foods from the Clorox bath, place them in clear water for ten minutes, and rinse. Dry all foods thoroughly and store.

FOOD GROUP	BATHING TIME
Leafy vegetables	15 minutes
Root, thick-skinned, or fibrous veggies	30 minutes
Thin-skinned fruits, such as berries, plums, peaches, and apricots	30 minutes
Thick-skinned fruits, such as citrus, bananas, and apples	30 minutes
Poultry, fish, meat, and eggs	20 minutes

Please do not place ground meat in the bath, but frozen meat can be thawed in a Clorox bath, allowing about twenty minutes for up to 5 pounds of meat.

Of course, you can always use apple cider vinegar or ¾ cup of 3% hydrogen peroxide in place of the Clorox. However, Dr. Parcells' lifetime of research suggested that the detoxifying results will be far from the same.

CHAPTER

10 Fat Flush Recipes

The basic Fat Flush recipes are quick and easy to prepare. Just ask the individuals who inspired them—my clients, readers, and Fat Flush iVillage community members. Like most of us, these Fat Flushers juggle family and career, so they simply don't have the time or energy to fuss with meals. In fact, according to the Wirthlin Women's Health Issues Survey of 1999, when racing against the clock, cooking is often the first thing to go by the wayside. This is why these recipes were created with the "less is definitely more" philosophy in mind.

But don't let this fool you. These recipes are big on flavor, especially with all the Fat Flushing herbs and spices. Almost all the recipes can be used in all phases of the plan—with the exception of the Vegetable Frittata and the Fruity Fruit Sorbet, marked with three asterisks (***), indicating that they are part of only phase 3.

Before you head for the kitchen, here are some helpful tips. When making your Fat Flush meals, avoid all aluminum-containing pots, pans, and foil. Food (especially acid-based foods) cooked in these utensils or wrapped in foil can leach the aluminum out, contributing to additional dietary aluminum. Aluminum hampers the body's use of calcium, magnesium, and phosphorus—those bone-building essentials. Instead of foil, I recommend Beyond Gourmet unbleached parchment paper, which is great for roasting vegetables and for *en papillote* oven cooking. You should be able to find it in most health food stores. If you must freeze or refrigerate food in aluminum foil, first wrap it in waxed paper so that the aluminum cannot leach into your food.

Preferable cookware includes high-quality stainless steel, cast iron (an especially good choice for anemics), enamel-coated iron, Corning Ware, Pyrex, and glass. I use the Royal Prestige electric frying pan for all of my Fat Flush Plan meals. The Royal Prestige is made of the highest surgical grade of stainless steel and uses a vacuum-sealed, minimum-moisture method so that food cooks without any added fat or vitamin-depleting water. I use a small amount of the vegetable, chicken, or beef broth in the pan for cooking virtually everything, even eggs.

When it comes to produce, fresh is always best—but frozen runs a close second. Many veggies and fruits are frozen at the peak of ripeness, so they usually have a lot of flavor. If using canned vegetables and fruits, be sure to drain the veggies well because the juices have added salt.

BREAKFAST

Fruit Smoothie

This is a refreshingly simple—and nutritious—way to start each day. Smoothies undoubtedly will become your staple fast-food breakfast. They are a quick and easy way to get your daily dose of flaxseed oil. If you are in phase 3, you also can choose from half of a banana, a small kiwi, or ½ cup of melon chunks for your fruit selection.

1 cup fresh or frozen fruit (strawberries, raspberries, blueberries, or frozen peaches or 1 fresh peach)
1 scoop or 2 heaping tablespoons protein powder
8 ounces cran-water or plain filtered water
1 tablespoon flaxseed oil
¼ teaspoon Stevia Plus to taste (optional)

- Place all ingredients in a blender.
- Blend until rich and creamy, approximately 2–3 minutes.

Makes 1 serving.

Breakfast Egg Fu Yung

Got five minutes? Whip up this tasty egg dish to start your day off right. A complete source of protein, eggs are loaded with key nutrients, such as vitamins, minerals, amino acids, and antioxidants, as well as the cholesterol-lowering phosphatidylcholine. You can even enhance the taste by topping it with a bit of Fat Flush Catsup (recipe in the "Condiment" section).

1 cup mushrooms, thinly sliced
1 garlic clove, diced
1 tablespoon no-salt-added chicken broth
½ cup mung bean sprouts
2 eggs, beaten with water
⅛ teaspoon cayenne pepper

- Cook mushrooms in broth over medium heat in a nonstick skillet.
- Add bean sprouts and garlic and sauté briefly.
- Pour eggs over mushrooms and sprouts.
- Cook over low heat until firm.
- Sprinkle with cayenne pepper.

Makes 1 serving.

Weekend Turkey-and-Egg Bake

Pamper yourself on your day off! Savory Fat Flushing herbs and fibrous veggies give this dish some real pizzazz while keeping you on track with your weight loss goals. Fennel, dill, and garlic aid the digestive process, and parsley helps reduce water weight.

½ pound lean ground turkey
1 cup mushrooms, chopped
½ cup onion, chopped
½ cup red pepper, chopped
¼ teaspoon dill
¼ teaspoon fennel, crushed
1 garlic clove, minced
2 eggs, beaten
¼ cup fresh parsley, minced
2 medium tomatoes, thinly sliced

- Preheat oven to 350°F.
- In a large skillet, cook the turkey, mushrooms, onion, red pepper, dill, fennel, and garlic together until the turkey is done.
- Drain off liquid, and place the mixture into a pie plate. In a medium bowl, stir together eggs and parsley, and then spread them over the turkey mixture.
- Bake uncovered for 25–30 minutes or until the top is set.
- Garnish with a nice arrangement of tomato slices and enjoy!

Makes 4 servings.

Vegetable Frittata***

Gourmet taste—yet so easy to do. And it's even better with delicious phytonutrient-rich vegetables.

½ pound fresh or frozen asparagus spears, cut up
4 eggs
½ cup low-fat cottage cheese
1 teaspoon dried mustard
Olive oil spray coating
½ cup mushrooms, thinly sliced
¼ cup onions, chopped (optional)
½ tomato, thinly sliced

- Preheat oven to 400°F.
- Steam asparagus for about 5 minutes until tender; then set aside.
- Beat eggs in a medium bowl until foamy. Beat in cottage cheese and mustard; then set aside.

- Lightly spray an ovenproof skillet with olive oil coating.
- Add mushrooms and onions (optional), and then cook over medium heat until tender.
- Stir in asparagus pieces.
- Pour egg mixture over veggies, and cook over low heat for about 5 minutes or until it bubbles slightly.
- Bake uncovered for about 10 minutes or until set.
- Garnish with tomato slices.

Makes 2 servings.

LUNCH OR DINNER ENTRÉES

Basic Stir-Fry

Looking for a tasty no-fuss meal? This stir-fry is made to order. You can alternate your protein choices for a slight twist.

¼ cup no-salt-added chicken broth
1 pound chicken, shrimp, lamb, or lean beef (your choice)
2 cups mushrooms, thinly sliced
1 cup bamboo shoots
1 cup water chestnuts
1 cup broccoli florets
1 cup asparagus, coarsely chopped
1 carrot, thinly sliced
1 teaspoon ginger
¼ teaspoon cayenne pepper

- Heat broth in a nonstick skillet over medium-high heat.
- Add your protein choice, and cook until almost done.
- Add veggies and seasonings, cooking until tender.

Makes 4 servings.

Rose's Fat Flush Soup

Try this scrumptious standby for lunch or dinner. This full-bodied soup has been a lifesaver for many on-the-go Fat Flushers wanting a meal-in-one.

1 pound ground beef or turkey
16 ounces Muir Glen Tomato Puree
16 ounces filtered water
½ onion, chopped
1 cup spinach, chopped
1 cup green beans, chopped

2 garlic cloves, minced
½ medium green pepper, chopped
½ medium red pepper, chopped
1 stalk celery, chopped

- Brown meat in a skillet over medium heat until no longer pink.
- Drain fat.
- Place the browned meat, water, onion, spinach, green beans, garlic, green and red peppers, and celery in large pot.
- Cook over low-medium heat for about 1 hour.

Makes 4 servings.

Cold Fish Salad

A great make-ahead meal that keeps fresh for several days.

2 tablespoons no-salt-added broth of your choice
Juice of 3–4 small limes
1 pound orange roughy fillets
½ cup onion, chopped
¼ cup fresh jalapeños, chopped (optional)
¾ cup tomatoes, chopped
¼ cup fresh parsley, chopped
2 cups cooked mustard greens

- Heat broth in a nonstick skillet.
- Place fish in skillet and pour lime juice over it, cooking until the fish is opaque.
- Add onion, jalapeños (optional), tomatoes, and parsley and cook for 5 minutes.
- Transfer to a serving dish and refrigerate for at least 2 hours until chilled.
- Serve on a bed of mustard greens.

Makes 4 servings.

Warm Turkey and Spinach Salad

Mealtime doesn't get any easier than this. Enjoy this dish for a quickie lunch or dinner.

1 tablespoon no-salt-added chicken broth
1 garlic clove, minced
¼ cup onion, diced
½ cup mushrooms, thinly sliced
½ cup tomato, diced

4 ounces turkey breast
1 cup fresh spinach, raw

- Sauté garlic and onion in broth over medium-high heat in a nonstick skillet until transparent and soft.
- Add mushrooms, tomato, and turkey, making sure that the turkey is brown on both sides or until done.
- Serve over raw spinach with your favorite Fat Flush dressing drizzled on top.

Makes 1 serving.

Gingered Shrimp and Snow Pea Soup

Freshly made, mouth-watering soup in just 25 minutes.

4 cups no-salt-added vegetable broth
¼ cup fresh ginger, sliced
¼ to ½ teaspoon cayenne pepper
2 cups snow peas, trimmed
1 pound shrimp, peeled and deveined
1 lemon, cut into wedges
2 tablespoons fresh cilantro or parsley, chopped

- Place broth and ginger in a large pot, and cover and simmer over medium-high heat for 15 minutes.
- Strain out ginger and return broth to pan.
- Add cayenne pepper and snow peas, simmering covered for about 5 minutes.
- Add shrimp and cook until firm (about 3 minutes).
- Squeeze lemon wedges into individual soup bowls and garnish each with cilantro (or parsley).

Makes 4 servings.

Friendly Italian Wedding Soup

Enjoy this romantic specialty from the Mediterranean—Fat Flush style.

1 pound lean ground beef
2 tablespoons garlic, minced
2 teaspoons fresh parsley, chopped
¼ cup diced onion
4 cups no-salt-added beef broth
1 carrot, chopped

1 cup spinach, chopped, packed, and well drained
Fresh garlic, minced, for garnish

- Combine the beef, garlic, parsley, and onion together.
- Shape into ½-inch meatballs.
- Brown meatballs in a nonstick skillet over medium heat until cooked and set aside.
- Pour broth into a large pot, add chopped carrot, and bring to a boil.
- Reduce heat, add meatballs, and simmer covered for about 20 minutes.
- Add spinach and simmer for 15 minutes longer.
- Garnish with lots of fresh garlic.

Makes 4 servings.

Eggplant Delight

An appetizing blend of flavors your whole family will love.

1 tablespoon no-salt-added beef broth
½ cup diced onion
2 garlic cloves, minced
1 pound ground lamb
1 teaspoon cumin
1 teaspoon cinnamon
1 can (14.5 ounces) no-salt-added Muir Glen Diced Tomatoes
1 medium eggplant, oven roasted (see recipe for Baked Eggplant in the "Veggie Sides" section)

- Preheat oven to 375°F.
- Heat broth over medium heat in a nonstick skillet.
- Add onion and garlic, and sauté until soft.
- Remove mixture to a bowl, and return pan to heat.
- Place lamb in the pan, and cook until it just begins to brown.
- Add the cumin and cinnamon, stir well, and sauté until meat is browned.
- Add onion-garlic mixture and tomatoes, simmering until juices evaporate.
- In a glass baking dish, arrange alternating layers of eggplant slices and lamb.
- Bake for 10 minutes.

Makes 4 servings.

Southwestern Flank Steak

Here's a hearty meal that's packed with gusto—and great on the barbie!

2 tablespoons fresh lime juice
1 tablespoon no-salt-added beef broth
2 garlic cloves, crushed
¼ teaspoon cayenne pepper (to taste)
2 teaspoons cumin
1 pound flank steak, thinly sliced on the diagonal
1 tablespoon no-salt-added beef broth
1 red pepper, thinly sliced
1 onion, thinly sliced

- Combine the lime juice, beef broth, garlic, cayenne, and cumin in a small bowl.
- Rub mixture over steak, and then transfer the steak to a baking dish and refrigerate for about 2 hours.
- Heat broiler (or prepare outdoor grill), and cook steak to desired doneness (5 minutes per side for medium).
- Meanwhile, heat broth in a nonstick skillet, and toss in red pepper and onion, cooking over medium heat.
- Stir constantly until onion is golden brown.
- Top steak with onion mixture and serve.

Makes 4 servings.

Grilled Lamb Chops with Cinnamon and Coriander

Who needs to eat out? These chops are lightly scented with savory Fat Flushing herbs that not only tickle your palate but also help rev up your metabolism and steady your blood sugar levels.

1 pound of lamb chops
2 tablespoons filtered water
1 tablespoon ground cinnamon
1 tablespoon ground coriander

- Preheat grill or broiler.
- Brush lamb with filtered water, and rub with cinnamon and coriander.
- Grill over medium heat, turning occasionally, about 20 minutes until done.

Makes 4 servings.

Shrimp Creole

You don't have to live in New Orleans to cook up a tantalizing Fat Flush–style Creole dish. This recipe uses colorful phytonutrients and thermogenic herbs to entice your senses—and help you shed those pounds.

4 tablespoons no-salt-added vegetable broth
3 green onions, white parts, thinly sliced
½ cup celery, thinly sliced
½ green pepper, diced
½ red pepper, diced
2 garlic cloves, minced
1 can (14.5 ounces) no-salt-added Muir Glen Tomato Sauce
½ cup filtered water
1 teaspoon fresh parsley, chopped
⅛ teaspoon cayenne pepper
8 ounces shrimp, peeled and deveined

- Warm broth in a nonstick skillet over low-medium heat.
- Add the green onions, celery, green and red pepper, and garlic and sauté until tender.
- Add the tomato sauce, water, parsley, and cayenne and simmer uncovered for 20 minutes.
- Toss in shrimp and stir. Heat to boiling. Reduce heat to low and cover, letting dish simmer 15–20 minutes or until shrimp are done.

Makes 2 servings.

Parsley and Dill Snapper Fillets

Make any night special with this tempting, easy-to-prepare dinner. Try it with your favorite fish, such as halibut, orange roughy, or sole.

1 pound red snapper (or fish of your choice)
½ cup no-salt-added vegetable broth
2 tablespoons parsley, minced
1 tablespoon shallots, minced
1 tablespoon fresh dill
¼ cup fresh lemon juice

- Preheat oven to 300°F.
- Arrange red snapper in the center of a baking dish, and add the broth, parsley, shallots, and dill.
- Place dish in oven, and roast until snapper is opaque in center, about 15–25 minutes.
- Transfer fish to serving dish.
- Add lemon juice to pan drippings, and then pour over fish.

Makes 4 servings.

Yummy Meatloaf

Can something this simple be this good and help you lose weight? You bet!

4 ounces meat (ground beef, veal, or turkey)
¼ cup spinach, chopped
¼ cup onion, diced
1 garlic clove, minced
⅛ teaspoon cayenne pepper
1 teaspoon fresh parsley, chopped
1 tablespoon no-salt-added Muir Glen Tomato Sauce

- Preheat oven to 400°F.
- Place the meat, spinach, onion, garlic, cayenne, and parsley in the bowl of a food processor and blend.
- Press into a mini–loaf pan and glaze the top with the tomato sauce.
- Bake for approximately 30 minutes.

Makes 1 serving.

Cumin Sautéed Scallops

For lunch or dinner, these tasty scallops will hit the spot. They burst with the unforgettable taste of scallion, garlic, and cumin.

4 tablespoons no-salt-added vegetable broth
2 scallions, minced
2 garlic cloves, minced
¼ teaspoon cumin
4 ounces scallops, trimmed and rinsed

- Heat broth in a nonstick skillet over medium heat.
- Add the scallions, garlic, and cumin and sauté for about 1 minute.
- Add the scallops and sauté until opaque.
- Remove the scallops from the skillet onto a plate and sprinkle with additional cumin, if desired.

Makes 1 serving.

Chicken-and-Cabbage Supreme

Think you've had it with chicken? Think again. The red pepper–cabbage combination gives this bird a whole new Fat Flushing attitude.

2 tablespoons no-salt-added chicken broth
1 pound boneless, skinless chicken, cut into 1-inch cubes
1 large onion, thinly sliced

4 garlic cloves, minced
1 large red pepper, cut lengthwise into ½-inch-thick slices
1 can (14.5 ounces) Muir Glen Whole Tomatoes, rinsed
½ cup Muir Glen Tomato Puree
1 stalk celery, cut into ½-inch-thick slices
1 small head of cabbage, shredded

- Cook chicken in broth over medium-high heat until cooked through.
- Add the onion, garlic, red pepper, tomatoes, and puree, bringing the mixture to a boil.
- Simmer covered for about 15 minutes.
- Add the celery and cabbage.
- Cover and simmer until cabbage is soft.

Makes 4 servings.

Braised Salmon

Aromatic herbs and spices make this omega-3–rich fish the catch of the day.

4 ounces salmon
½ can (7 ounces) Muir Glen Stewed Tomatoes, rinsed
¼ cup Muir Glen Tomato Puree
5 garlic cloves, roasted (see recipe below)
½ scallion, thinly sliced
1 large mushroom, thinly sliced
1 teaspoon coriander
1 tablespoon fresh lemon juice
1 tablespoon fresh parsley, chopped, for garnish

- Place salmon skin side down in a nonstick skillet.
- Add the tomatoes, tomato purée, garlic, scallion, mushroom, and coriander and cover.
- Simmer over medium heat for about 15 minutes.
- When salmon is done, remove from skillet onto plate, drizzling with lemon juice and garnishing with parsley.

Makes 1 serving.

Tomato-Herb Veal

Middle of the week blahs? Here's a delightful change of pace. If veal isn't your thing, try the recipe with sirloin steak.

¼ cup onion, chopped
1 garlic clove, minced

2 tablespoons filtered water
1 can (14.5 ounces) no-salt-added Muir Glen Diced Tomatoes
1 tablespoon fresh parsley, chopped
2 tablespoons no-salt-added beef broth
1 pound boneless veal leg round or sirloin steak, cut ¼ inch thick with fat trimmed off

- Sauté onion and garlic in water in a medium saucepan over medium heat until the onion is soft and the garlic is transparent.
- Stir in tomatoes and parsley, bring to a boil, and reduce heat.
- Cook uncovered for 10 minutes, then set aside.
- Heat broth in another skillet over medium-high heat, and then add meat, cooking to desired doneness.
- Remove meat from the skillet onto a plate.
- Spoon tomato-herb sauce over meat and serve.

Makes 4 servings.

Cider Turkey with Mushrooms

Quick and zesty. A great pick-me-up on those hurried Fat Flush days.

1 pound skinless turkey, cut into 1-inch cubes
2 tablespoons no-salt-added chicken broth
4 cups mushrooms, sliced
¼ cup red pepper, diced (optional)
¼ cup apple cider vinegar
⅛ cup fresh parsley, chopped, for garnish

- Cook turkey in broth in a nonstick skillet over medium-high heat until the turkey is cooked through.
- Add mushrooms, red pepper (optional), and vinegar, cooking until soft.
- Remove from the skillet onto a plate.
- Garnish with fresh parsley.

Makes 4 servings.

Chicken Kabob

Even the kids will eat their veggies with this dish.

1 pound skinless chicken, cut into 1-inch cubes
2 cups zucchini, cubed
2 cups yellow squash, cubed
2 cups red pepper, cubed

½ pound button mushrooms
Lemon wedges, for garnish

- Preheat grill or broiler.
- Alternate chicken and vegetable cubes on skewers.
- Grill for about 15–20 minutes, turning at least once, until chicken is cooked through.
- Remove from the grill onto a serving platter.
- Garnish with lemon and serve.

Makes 4 servings.

Lamb Stir-Fry

Who doesn't love a good stir-fry? This one breaks the ho-hum mold, tossing lean lamb with Fat Flushing herbs and spices.

¼ cup green onion, sliced
¼ cup fresh parsley, chopped
1½ tablespoons lemon juice
1 teaspoon dried mustard
1 pound lean boneless lamb, cut into 1-inch cubes
2 tablespoons no-salt-added beef broth
1 garlic clove, minced
1 green or red pepper, thinly sliced
2 tablespoons no-salt-added beef broth

- In a medium bowl, combine onion, parsley, lemon juice, and dried mustard.
- Stir in lamb chunks, coating them thoroughly, and set aside.
- Heat broth in a nonstick skillet over medium heat.
- Add garlic and peppers, sautéing for about 2–3 minutes over medium heat.
- Take out and set aside.
- Heat remaining broth in the skillet, adding the lamb mixture.
- Cook until lamb is cooked through.
- Mix the garlic and peppers with the lamb mixture.
- Heat through.
- Remove stir-fry from the skillet to a plate and serve.

Makes 4 servings.

HOMEMADE BROTHS AND EASY SOUPS

If you can't find salt-free store-bought vegetable, chicken, and beef broths, you can always make your own, and even more nutritiously at that. The key is to use bones with your homemade broth and add a couple of tablespoons of apple cider vinegar. This will up the calcium content because the vinegar actually helps leach calcium from the bones. And whenever possible, I would suggest using free-range, hormone- and antibiotic-free chicken or beef rather than commercially raised chicken or beef.

These broths can be used at every phase of the Fat Flush Plan for sautéing veggies, scrambling eggs, or basting any protein dish.

Freeze broths in an ice cube tray for convenient future use. Each "broth ice cube" is approximately 1 tablespoon of broth.

1-2-3 Vegetable Broth

Enhance any mealtime with this delicate brew.

2 quarts filtered water
1 large onion, cut in 1-inch pieces
3 stalks celery, cut in 1-inch pieces
1 bunch green onion, chopped
8 cloves garlic, minced
8 sprigs fresh parsley
8 ounces mushrooms, cut in ½-inch slices
2 bay leaves

- Place all ingredients in a large stockpot, and bring to a boil.
- Lower heat and simmer uncovered for about 1 hour.
- Strain, and discard vegetables.
- Refrigerate and use within 3 days or freeze.

Makes 4 servings.

1-2-3 Chicken Broth

A nutritious way to bolster the flavor of your Fat Flush recipes.

2 quarts filtered water
3 pounds chicken pieces with the bones
3 tablespoons cider vinegar
1 large onion, cut in 1-inch pieces
3 stalks celery, cut in 1-inch pieces
4 sprigs fresh parsley
2 bay leaves

- Place all ingredients in a large pot, and bring to a boil.
- Reduce heat, cover, and simmer for about 45 minutes or until the chicken is done.
- Strain, and discard vegetables and bones; save the chicken for another recipe.
- Refrigerate and use within 3 days or freeze.

Makes 4 servings.

1-2-3 Beef Broth

A healthy and hearty base for any Fat Flush meal.

3 pounds beef shank
1 large onion, cut in 1-inch pieces
2 quarts filtered water
3 tablespoons apple cider vinegar
3 stalks celery, cut in 1-inch pieces
4 sprigs fresh parsley
4 garlic cloves, minced
2 bay leaves

- Preheat oven to 450°F.
- Place bones and onions in a roasting pan.
- Bake for 30 minutes or until bones are browned.
- Remove from oven.
- Place bones and onions in a large stockpot.
- Add water, vinegar, celery, parsley, garlic, and bay leaves to the stockpot, and bring to a boil.
- Reduce heat, cover, and simmer for 3 hours.
- Strain, and discard vegetables and bones; save the meat for another recipe.
- Refrigerate and use within 3 days or freeze.

Makes 4 servings.

Egg Drop–Cilantro Soup

East meets the Southwest. Here's a unique Fat Flush combo that also gets that slimming protein into your diet.

4 cups no-salt-added chicken broth
2 eggs, well beaten
¼ cup cilantro, chopped, for garnish

- Place broth in a large pot and bring to a boil over medium-high heat.
- In a small bowl, beat eggs with a fork.
- Gradually stir the beaten eggs into the broth.
- Reduce heat, stirring continuously with a fork until the egg stands out from the stock.
- Remove from heat, and pour into bowls.
- Garnish with cilantro and serve immediately.

Makes 4 servings.

VEGGIE SIDES

Roasted Veggie Medley

Now here's a no-fuss side dish you'll definitely want to try. The veggies will really taste great because the broth seals in the flavor. Try eggplant, zucchini, or maybe even yellow squash. And if you haven't met your daily flaxseed oil requirement, drizzle the remaining amount over the veggies. Tasty!

½ cup red bell pepper, cut into strips
½ cup yellow bell pepper, cut into strips
½ cup onion, thinly sliced
½ cup mushrooms, thinly sliced
2 tablespoons no-salt-added broth of your choice

- Place veggies in a baking dish.
- Brush and blend with broth.
- Broil for about 10 minutes.

Makes 1 serving.

Zesty Coleslaw

Want a little crunch—and a whole lot of zing? Here it is. For an extra treat, you may want to save some of your daily flaxseed oil requirement to drizzle over your slaw.

1 cup shredded green cabbage
½ cup shredded red cabbage
½ cup jícama, peeled and grated
½ small green pepper, coarsely chopped
½ small red pepper, coarsely chopped
½ small onion, coarsely chopped
1 small stalk celery, chopped

Dressing:
½ cup apple cider vinegar
½ teaspoon garlic, minced
½ teaspoon Stevia Plus (optional)
½ teaspoon cayenne pepper (optional)

- Combine the cabbage, jícama, peppers, onion, and celery in a large serving bowl.
- In another bowl, create the dressing by stirring the vinegar, garlic, and (optional) Stevia Plus and cayenne pepper until well blended.
- Add the dressing to the vegetable mixture and toss lightly.
- Cover and refrigerate for at least 1 hour before serving.

Makes 4 servings.

Baked Eggplant

Want a savory vegetable dish that's loaded with fiber and low in calories? This easy eggplant is one of Fat Flushers' top choices every time.

¼ cup no-salt-added broth (beef, chicken, or vegetable)
1 medium eggplant, cut into ½-inch slices
Juice of 1 lemon

- Preheat oven to 425°F.
- Pour the broth into a roasting pan.
- Place the eggplant slices into the pan, lightly coating them on both sides with the broth.
- Bake for 10 minutes.
- Turn eggplant slices over, and bake for another 10 minutes.
- Add lemon juice and let set for a few minutes.

Makes 4 servings.

Warm Asparagus and Mushrooms

This is one flavorful veggie blend your whole family will love. And it's good for them too. Asparagus has a marvelous cleansing effect on the kidneys and bladder, and mushrooms are rich in the calming B vitamins.

1 pound asparagus spears, cut into 1-inch pieces
1 tablespoon no-salt-added vegetable broth
4 cups mushrooms, thinly sliced
½ cup onion, chopped
1 tablespoon garlic, minced

¼ cup fresh lemon juice
2–4 tablespoons flaxseed oil

- Prepare fresh asparagus by gently bending the stalk until it snaps.
- Discard the bottom half and slice the rest on the diagonal.
- Steam the asparagus for about 5-6 minutes until crisp but tender.
- Set aside.
- Heat the broth, mushrooms, onion, and garlic in a nonstick skillet, cooking until soft.
- Add the asparagus, and drizzle with lemon juice.
- Heat the asparagus through over low-medium heat.
- Remove from the skillet to a serving platter and allow to cool.
- Drizzle ½ to 1 tablespoon flaxseed oil over each serving at room temperature.

Makes 4 servings.

Savory Spaghetti Squash

Here's a delicious way to blend those Fat Flushing nutrients with the thermogenic power of cinnamon. When selecting your smooth, watermelon-shaped squash, look for one that has a hard, deep-colored rind.

1 spaghetti squash
2 large garlic cloves, minced
½ teaspoon cinnamon
1–2 tablespoons flaxseed oil

- Cut squash in half, and scoop out the seeds.
- Place the squash halves on a nonstick baking sheet, cut side down.
- Bake at 375°F for 30 minutes.
- With a fork, separate the spaghetti pulp from the skin, and place the pulp in a serving dish.
- Sprinkle on garlic, cinnamon, and oil, and toss lightly.

Makes 4 servings.

Roasted Garlic

Forget those fancy restaurants—you can roast your own garlic easily at home. Do it a couple of times a week, and then keep it in the fridge for at least 3-4 days for whenever you want to dress up a meal or side dish.

Garlic heads, as many as desired

- Preheat oven to 350°F.
- Wrap garlic head(s) in parchment paper.
- Place in oven for about 45 minutes.

Marinated Artichoke Salad

This fat-burning number bursts with flavor and eye appeal!

2 cans (13–15 ounces) artichokes hearts packed in water (or 2 cups filtered water plus 4 fresh artichoke hearts)
1 garlic clove, minced
4 tablespoons flaxseed oil
¼ cup fresh lemon juice
1½ tablespoons apple cider vinegar
½ teaspoon cayenne pepper
Tricolored greens, for garnish

- Drain the (canned) artichoke hearts, and rinse well with water.
- Place 4 artichoke hearts in a large bowl, and mash with the garlic.
- Stir in the flaxseed oil, lemon juice, vinegar, and cayenne, and mix well.
- Quarter the remaining hearts, and mix well with the dressing.
- Refrigerate at least 1 hour.
- Arrange on bed of greens and serve.

Makes 4 servings.

SALAD DRESSINGS

Refreshing Salad Dressing

In the mood for a little zing? Try this on a bed of lettuce and cut-up vegetables.

4 tablespoons flaxseed oil
3 tablespoons apple cider vinegar
3 tablespoons fresh lemon juice

- Put all ingredients in a small covered jar, and shake vigorously for 30 seconds.

Makes 4 servings.

Lime-Scented Flax Dressing

Perfect for a refreshing pick-me-up.

4 tablespoons flaxseed oil
4 tablespoons fresh lime juice
2 cloves garlic, minced
¼ teaspoon cayenne pepper

- Put all ingredients in a small covered jar, and shake vigorously for 30 seconds.

Makes 4 servings.

CONDIMENTS

Fat Flush Catsup

All of the flavor—but none of the guilt.

2 tablespoons Muir Glen Tomato Puree
1½ teaspoons apple cider vinegar
⅛ teaspoon Stevia Plus
½ teaspoon garlic, finely minced
Pinch of cayenne (optional)

- Place all ingredients in a small bowl, and stir well with a wire whisk.

Makes 1 serving.

Fat Flush Cocktail Sauce

Delicious way to complement shrimp or other fish favorites.

Fat Flush Catsup (recipe above)
1 teaspoon fresh lemon or lime juice
¼ teaspoon dried mustard
1 teaspoon fresh cilantro, chopped finely
3 pinches cayenne pepper, to taste

- Prepare the Fat Flush Catsup as directed.
- Add the lemon (or lime) juice, dried mustard, cilantro, and cayenne pepper.
- Mix well with a wire whisk.

Makes 1 serving.

Homemade Salsa

This Fat Flushing dip will have your whole family shouting, "Olé!" You can make it in a snap and dip strips of your favorite veggies in it.

1 to 2 fresh small jalapeño peppers, minced (optional)
⅛ cup cilantro, finely minced
¼ cup green pepper, finely diced
2 garlic cloves, finely minced
1 can (14.5 ounces) no-salt-added Muir Glen Diced Tomatoes, drained
Juice of half a lime
6 green onions (white parts only), finely diced
2 tablespoons apple cider vinegar

- Blend all ingredients together.
- Refrigerate a few hours or overnight.

Makes 4 servings.

SNACKS

Fat Flush "Deviled" Eggs

There's nothing bad about these eggs! They're loaded with slimming omega-3 and dressed with Fat Flushing herbs.

2 eggs, hard-boiled
½ tablespoon flaxseed oil
½ teaspoon apple cider vinegar
¼ teaspoon dried mustard
½ teaspoon green onion (white part), finely minced
¼ to ½ teaspoon finely minced garlic (to taste)
Pinch of cayenne pepper (optional)
Sprigs of fresh dill and parsley, for garnish

- Cool the hard-boiled eggs under cold water.
- Peel eggs, and cut in half lengthwise.
- Remove the yolks, and put them in a small bowl.
- Add oil, vinegar, onion, garlic, and mustard to yolks, and mix thoroughly. Scoop the yolk mixture with a spoon, and use it to fill the egg halves.
- Top with dill and parsley.

Makes 1 to 2 servings.

TREATS

Fruity Fruit Sorbet***

Once you've graduated to the Lifestyle Eating Plan, treat yourself to this delightful dessert. It's allowed only in phase 3 because, unlike the blended fruits, protein powder, and flaxseed oil in the breakfast smoothies, this recipe is really pure fruit, without the balancing nutrition of the protein and oil to level out blood sugar. Puréeing breaks down the fiber in fruits, which also can affect blood sugar levels by concentrating the sugars.

½ cup strawberries, halved
½ cup raspberries
1 teaspoon fresh lemon juice (optional)
¼ to ½ teaspoon Stevia Plus (optional to taste if fruit is not sweet enough)

- Place all ingredients in a food processor or blender and purée until smooth.
- Freeze until firm (about 3–4 hours only).

Makes 1 serving.

TIME-SAVING TIP | **Start with partially thawed frozen fruit so that you can eat your sorbet immediately.**

I love that I can maintain the Lifestyle Eating Plan without starving or going off the deep end with cravings! I have found that I enjoy the tastes of proteins and veggies without all the salt and trans fats I used before. I like the plan's more natural approach, and feel much better cutting out all the processed foods and excess carbs. And I am really happy to be able to eat eggs again. I have been avoiding them for years because of high cholesterol. I don't even miss my coffee in the morning. I just stick to hot water with lemon or healthy tea.

—*BARB K.*

FAT FLUSH SEASONING SAVVY

No doubt you have noticed that many of the menus and recipes contain the special Fat Flushing culinary herbs and spices, which can turn simple dishes into exotic entrées and sides. Cayenne, cumin, parsley, cilantro, dill, anise, fennel, bay leaves, ginger, cloves, coriander, cinnamon, mustard, and apple cider vinegar are not just your everyday flavoring favorites; they are essential to the Fat Flushing strategy because they rev up the metabolism, help remove excess fluid from tissues, and control cravings. Here are some examples of how I like to use these Fat Flushing seasonings to spice up my life. Give them a try.

FOOD	HERBS AND SPICES
Fish	Dill, fennel, ginger
Beef	Cumin, garlic, cloves
Lamb	Cinnamon, garlic, cloves
Poultry	Mustard, garlic, cayenne
Eggs	Parsley, cumin, mustard
Soups	Bay leaf, parsley, dill
Cabbage	Anise, ginger, apple cider vinegar
Cucumber	Dill, apple cider vinegar, parsley
Greens	Garlic, apple cider vinegar, dill
Squash	Cinnamon, cloves, ginger

For a more cosmopolitan flavor, you can rub the following dry blends directly on your meat, fish, lamb, or poultry and cook:

ASIAN: ⅛ cup ground ginger, 1 tablespoon dried mustard, 1 minced garlic clove, and 1 teaspoon chopped onion

TEX-MEX: 2 tablespoons cumin, 1 teaspoon coriander, ½ teaspoon cayenne, and ½ teaspoon cinnamon

MOROCCAN: ½ cup chopped onion, 2 minced garlic cloves, 2 teaspoons cumin and coriander, ¼ teaspoon cayenne pepper

MAKING YOUR FAVORITE RECIPES FAT FLUSH FRIENDLY FOR LIFESTYLE EATING

Here are some tips on how to modify recipe ingredients for your old-time favorites or holiday specialties to make them Fat Flush friendly for the Lifestyle phase of the program. Name brands and/or contact information can be found in Chapter 9. I have found many tasty ways to cut out the trans fats, sugar, salt, refined carbohydrates, and gluten from my recipes without sacrificing flavor for your family's favorite recipes. The following chart provides some easy-to-use tips for replacing traditional recipe ingredients. I guarantee that taste will not be sacrificed by these substitutions—in fact, it is enhanced. Try them out for yourself. Even your company won't know the difference.

I'm a Feng Shui consultant and own my own company. One Saturday morning, while driving, I heard about the Fat Flush Plan on a radio show. At that time I was feeling particularly bloated, fat, and disgusted with myself. I was sixty-two years old and not only had the potbelly, but also a roll of fat on top of it. At 5'7" I was pushing 160 pounds for the first time in my life. I was starting to look in plus size shops for clothes, and thought, "No, I can't do this." I decided to give the plan a try. Suddenly, I began dropping the weight and feeling really wonderful. I'm down to 136 pounds, having lost around 24 pounds total. Now I even feel comfortable in a bathing suit.

After the Fat Flush, my eating habits changed—and it really wasn't difficult. I had always loved pasta and bread, but found that cutting those things out made a world of difference in my weight loss.

I'd tried other diets like most people, but this is the first time I tried one that actually worked. Now when I make food choices, I remember the Fat Flush principles, like using flaxseed oil and drinking cranberry juice. When I went on vacation recently, I ate too much. So when I got back home, I did a five-day Fat Flush and felt good again. I'm grateful for the tools given to me by the Fat Flush program, and will use them whenever I need to get back on track.

—IRENE AVERELL

WHEN THE RECIPE CALLS FOR:	USE THIS FAT FLUSH INGREDIENT INSTEAD:
1 tablespoon of margarine, cooking oil, or butter	3 tablespoons ground flaxseed. Your baked goods will brown more quickly with flax, so either shorten the baking time or lower oven temperature by 25°F.
Sugar	Use 1 packet Stevia Plus for every 2 teaspoons of sugar. Or use aromatic crushed seeds such as fennel, cardamom, anise, caraway, or coriander.
1 cup whole or skim milk	2 heaping tablespoons high-protein whey powder plus 1 cup filtered water.
Hot pepper sauce	Dash of cayenne.
1 teaspoon dried herbs	1 tablespoon fresh herbs.
1 teaspoon salt	1 teaspoon Cardia Salt.
1 ounce or square of unsweetened baking chocolate	3 tablespoons of carob powder plus 1 tablespoon of filtered water and 1 tablespoon rice bran oil.
1 tablespoon cocoa	1 tablespoon carob powder.
2 tablespoons margarine mixed with1 tablespoon flour for sauce and soup thickeners	2 tablespoons arrowroot or kudzu found in health food stores. Arrowroot adds calcium to foods, whereas kudzu is high in iron. Or use egg yolks to thicken sauces or puréed cauliflower for soups.
1 cup whole grain flour for baking	Take 2 tablespoons out of 1 cup of flour and replace it with 2 tablespoons of flax meal. Reduce the oil in the recipe by 2 teaspoons for every 2 tablespoons of the flax meal. Bake for a shorter time or lower the heat by 25°F.
1 egg	1 omega-3–enriched egg. (Note: If you're allergic to eggs, blend 1 tablespoon ground flax with 3 tablespoons of water and let stand for a couple of minutes.)
Gelatin	Agar-agar, a seaweed gelatin available in health food stores replaces animal-based gelatin. Agar-agar provides added fiber and lubrication in the intestinal tract by absorbing moisture.
Baking powder, regular (contains aluminum)	Equal amounts of aluminum-free baking powder, low-sodium and grain-free.
Breading and frying	Poach in broth, water, or wine, and then bake in a covered dish to retain moisture.

OTHER COOKING HELP

Here are some quick facts on equivalent measurements to help you with Fat Flush recipes and with figuring out your weekly shopping list.

Dry and Liquid Equivalents

1 teaspoon or less	=	a pinch
3 teaspoons	=	1 tablespoon
4 tablespoons	=	¼ cup
5⅓ tablespoons	=	⅓ cup
8 tablespoons	=	½ cup
10⅔ tablespoons	=	⅔ cup
16 tablespoons	=	1 cup
2 cups	=	1 pint
4 cups	=	1 quart
2 pints	=	1 quart
4 quarts	=	1 gallon

1 cup chopped onion	=	1 large onion
1 cup chopped sweet pepper	=	1 large pepper
1 cup chopped tomato	=	1 large tomato
½ cup chopped tomato	=	2 plum tomatoes
½ cup diced celery	=	1 large stalk
3 tablespoons sliced scallion	=	1 large scallion
1 teaspoon chopped garlic	=	1 large clove
3 tablespoons lemon juice	=	juice of 1 medium lemon
2 tablespoons lime juice	=	juice of 1 lime
1 tablespoon fresh herb	=	1 teaspoon dried herb
1 cup sliced mushrooms	=	6 to 8 medium mushrooms
¼ teaspoon Stevia Plus	=	1 packet Stevia Plus

CHAPTER

11 Because You Asked

Whether I'm on a book tour, speaking before an audience, doing a radio show, or chatting on the iVillage.com interactive board, I always look forward to hearing from men and women around the world. In fact, getting to speak with them firsthand is perhaps the most enjoyable part of my profession. I always love to hear how people are inspired by the Fat Flush Plan, how sound nutrition is revitalizing their lives, and how I can assist them even more by answering their questions.

Since there tends to be a common thread in their concerns, I thought you might benefit from reading through some of the most frequently asked questions about the Fat Flush Plan.

AGES, STAGES, AND GENDER

Is there an age limit for Fat Flush?

YES AND NO. I believe that the first two phases of the program are too stringent for children under age 12; however, phase 3 is a healthy option. Regardless of their age, your children definitely can benefit from adding the right fats to their current dietary regimen whether they are on the plan or not! In fact, the most remarkable news about omega-3–rich oils (such as flaxseed and fish oils) is their dramatic effect on children. Many clinical studies have shown how low brain chemistry levels of these essential fatty acids are connected with a multitude of neurological and psychological symptoms, including attention deficit hyperactivity disorder (ADHD), depression, and violent behavior. Adding from 2 teaspoons to 1 tablespoon of flaxseed oil to your child's cereal or pancake toppings is one of the best oil changes you can make. In fact, it is a great idea to make such changes for the whole family as well.

And speaking of oil changes, your teenage daughter can benefit too. By taking the gamma-linolenic acid (GLA)–rich evening primrose oil for two weeks before her period, your daughter can say goodbye to premenstrual syndrome (PMS)–related headaches, irritability, bloating, cramping, and breast tenderness. Your children will quickly experience—even faster than you—how the right fats are a friend, not a foe.

What about pregnant or breastfeeding women—can they be on the Fat Flush Plan?

There are times in a woman's life cycle that demand optimal nutritional support and additional calories. Pregnancy and breastfeeding are definitely two such times.

A pregnant woman should be focused on gaining weight—*not* losing or maintaining weight—which are the primary goals of each phase of the plan. In fact, in the second and third trimesters of pregnancy, a woman needs at least 300 extra calories each day and she needs another 500 extra calories each day while breastfeeding. For a healthy pregnancy, doctors typically recommend that most women gain between 25 and 30 pounds. If a woman is underweight, gaining 28 to 40 pounds is suggested; if overweight, adding 15 to 25 pounds is recommended.

Having said that, phase 3 can be used as a foundational eating program for pregnant or breastfeeding women, utilizing the full array of servings in every food category as a baseline—and even adding on servings in each category if weight gain is not sufficient or the person is still hungry. The only dietary change, based upon the recommendation of the Food and Drug Administration (FDA), would be to limit fish intake to only 12 ounces per week and completely eliminate larger fish such as shark, swordfish, tilefish, and king mackerel while pregnant or breastfeeding. These fish are more likely to be contaminated with toxic mercury, and exposure to mercury can result in neurological problems and learning deficits in children. Plus, the recommended weight loss supplements, with the exception of a daily multiple vitamin with extra folic acid, should be omitted at this time—especially those with herbal ingredients.

I highly recommend the initial two phases of the Fat Flush Plan after women give birth and/or stop breastfeeding for a safe body cleansing and weight loss regimen.

In addition to the flaxseed oil and GLA supplements, pregnant and breastfeeding women can supplement their diet with other essential fatty acids that can be integrated into phase 3 right away. The most important is docosahexaenoic acid (DHA), which is found in the fattier fish (such as salmon and sardines) and even in omega-3-enriched eggs. In capsule form, DHA is usually purified to remove polychlorinated biphenyls (PCBs) and heavy metals such as mercury and arsenic.

Since the human brain is composed of 60 percent fat and the most prevalent fat is DHA, this primary building block is absolutely essential for proper cognitive and visual development. Infants depend on mother's milk for their DHA. However, the DHA level in the breast milk of American women is the lowest in the world.

I always suggest that pregnant women take a dietary supplement containing 200 mg of DHA along with their prenatal supplements. Breastfeeding women can double this amount to 400 mg, which will benefit the baby and also the mother, by protecting against postpartum depression.

Mothers unable to breastfeed should consider adding 100 mg of DHA to each bottle of formula.

I recommend a DHA brand called Neuromins—available in health food stores—because these supplements are derived from algae (the fish's original source), making them acceptable to all vegetarians, even vegans.

Is there anything special a woman should do at certain stages of her life, such as perimenopause or menopause?

Yes, there is. Studies comparing Asian menopausal women with Western menopausal women showed the Asian women have a much easier transition and better overall health. One of the reasons may be their daily intake (from 45 to 100 mg) of the stabilizing phytoestrogens called isoflavones. Isoflavones are highly touted for relieving such symptoms as hot flashes, sweats, etc., caused by hormonal fluctuations. They are found most prevalently in soy, red clover, kudzu root, and lignans.

These isoflavones are accepted by human cell estrogen receptors, so they satisfy the body's estrogen needs and thereby relieve perimenopausal symptoms. As weak estrogenic mimics, these isoflavones also aid in stabilizing fluctuating estrogen and progesterone levels and reduce cholesterol while helping to maintain strong bones.

For menopausal Fat Flushing women, there are many elements of the daily routine that offer hormone-stabilizing benefits. The selection of ground flaxseeds in the Long Life Cocktail as well as the GLA provided by the evening primrose oil, borage, or black currant seed oil helps to balance mood swings, quell hot flashes and night sweats, and provide welcome lubrication for tissue dryness.

My husband wants to follow the Fat Flush Plan. What can he expect, and should men do anything differently?

Men typically lose from 8 to 16 pounds in phase 1. They have greater muscle mass than women—20 percent more, in fact. And having more lean muscle mass means that men have the ability to lose weight faster than women. Pound for pound, muscle can burn more calories than fat—giving men a built-in advantage (literally).

Men who follow the Fat Flush Plan usually make some personal adjustments to the plan. They typically jump from phase 1 to phase 3, because they need more fuel in the form of friendly carbs for their higher metabolism.

Also, some men also feel that they need more than 8 ounces of protein per day and increase portion sizes of meat, fish, and chicken by 2 ounces at lunch and at dinner. Many feel more comfortable if they double up on the whey protein powder in the morning.

Could my thyroid-related weight problem be tied to any other kind of hormonal imbalance?

Yes, especially if you are lacking natural progesterone and are estrogen-dominant (see Chapter 2). Synthetic estrogens in the form of birth control pills or hormone-replacement therapy (HRT) elevate sex hormone–binding globulin (SHBG), which can depress other hormones, including thyroid hormone. The resulting symptoms range from weight gain and fatigue to cold hands and feet as well as an inability to sweat. Estrogen and progesterone levels can be assessed through testing. You can also try using a cream with a natural form of progesterone , which is identical to what your body makes. Monitor the results over a three-month period by tracking your progress in your journal, noting your energy and overall well-being. If these improve on progesterone, then your thyroid-related weight problem is tied to estrogen dominance and progesterone deficit. (See Chapter 12.)

FAT FLUSH PROTOCOL

Do I really have to stick to the Fat Flush Plan exactly as described, or can I personalize it a bit?

You certainly can personalize the Fat Flush Plan to suit your own needs. The program is based on principles, not just on hard-and-fast dos and don'ts. Of course, I would like you to build your meals around as many Fat Flushing elements as possible to get the best results: the Long Life Cocktail, hot water and lemon, increased water, lean protein, low-glycemic-index fruits and vegetables, flaxseed oil, and GLA supplements. Each of these elements has specific fat-burning and diuretic properties.

One of the most common ways to personalize the phase 1 Fat Flush—especially for those who aren't willing to give up their heavy-duty workout routines—is to add in one or two friendly carbs (see Chapter 5) from the get-go. One slice of sprouted whole-grain bread (such as toasted Ezekiel 4:9—a delicious bread recommended and listed in Chapter 9) at breakfast and/or a half cup of peas or cooked carrots, winter squash, or sweet potato at night seem to satisfy Fat Flush athletes the most.

Is there a reason why flaxseed oil is taken with food and not alone?

Yes, there is. When you blend your flaxseed oil with other foods (such as using the oil in salad dressings or topping your veggies), it helps emulsify the oil, which ensures better absorption and therefore better use of the essential fatty acids the oil contains. In fact, the famed German biochemist Dr. Johanna Budwig, who did most of the early research on flax, always combined flaxseed oil, either with vegetables or in yogurt and no-heat recipes.

Can I cook with flaxseed oil and keep my flaxseed oil in the fridge?

You can't cook with flaxseed oil because it is a highly unsaturated oil, which means it is very sensitive to heat, air, and light and can go rancid if not treated properly. For these reasons, you also should keep it in the fridge. If you purchase the 8-ounce container, you will need to use it up in about three weeks.

If you live in a colder climate, however, you can store flaxseed oil in a cool, dark place rather than in the fridge during cooler weather. Flaxseed oil also can be stored in the freezer for up to one year.

I've heard that flaxseeds can be harmful—is this true?

Lignan-rich flaxseeds are safe in proper amounts. They do, however, contain a substance known as cyanogenic glycosides, as do lima beans, sweet potatoes, yams, and bamboo shoots. Cyanogenic glycosides metabolize into yet another substance, known as thiocyanate (SCN)—a chemical that has the potential, over time, of suppressing the thyroid's ability to take up sufficient iodine. This biochemical occurrence raises the risk of developing goiter.

There are two easy ways to avoid this problem. One is to consume a *maximum* of 3 or 4 tablespoons of ground-up flaxseeds per day. The other is to lightly bake or toast your flaxseeds, which deactivates and decomposes the cyanogenic glycosides but preserves the beneficial omega-3 properties. To toast them, you spread flaxseeds on a baking sheet or pan and then place it in a 250°F oven for fifteen to twenty minutes until the seeds are crispy. (*Please note:* Using any temperatures above 300°F will damage the seeds' oil and convert it into the unhealthy trans form.)

Flaxseed oil, on the other hand, is free of cyanogenic glycosides.

Why isn't canola oil on the Fat Flush Plan?

Canola oil, which means "Canadian oil," is not the most desirable source of essential fatty acids (such as the omega-3–rich flax and fish oils or the omega-6–rich GLA from evening primrose oil, borage oil, or black currant seed oil). Also, I am concerned that the majority of canola oil on the market today is highly refined and genetically engineered. This opens up a Pandora's box of dangers, including no long-term safety testing and unforeseen and unknown allergens.

Why do you limit certain herbs and spices?

On the first two phases of the Fat Flush Plan, you are concentrating on dropping pounds while cleansing your system. The selected herbs and spices in these initial phases are considered either thermogenic (which means they rev up the body's metabolic fires and jumpstart energy expenditure), diuretic, or helpful in carbohydrate metabolism and digestion.

Actually, though, the spices aren't limited in the sense that you can't have savory meals. There are plenty of tasty, thermogenic choices to spice up your life, including cayenne, dried mustard, ginger, and garlic. Besides providing flavor, these herbs and spices help with your weight loss and health goals: Bay leaves, cinnamon, cloves, and coriander help control insulin levels; parsley, cilantro, fennel, anise, and apple cider vinegar act as natural diuretics; dill, fennel, and anise aid digestion; and cumin helps protect against degenerative disease.

Since dairy isn't allowed in phase 1 or phase 2, how will I get enough calcium?

Not to worry. You'll get plenty with the bone-building green leafy veggies, which are used liberally in the menu plans. For instance, you'll enjoy kale, watercress, parsley, escarole, mesclun salad greens, dandelion greens, turnip greens, bok choy, arugula, chickory, endive, and broccoli.

Just to give you an example, a cup of milk has 300 mg of calcium. A cup of collard greens has 226 mg of calcium, a cup of turnip greens has 195 mg, and a cup of dandelion greens has 147 mg. And a cup of broccoli has around 250 mg of calcium. You'll be having lots of these calcium-rich greens at lunch and dinner. And sautéed in broth with 1 to 2 teaspoons of apple cider vinegar, they are really quite tasty.

The World Health Organization recommends just 450 mg of calcium per day, which is a far cry from the 800 to 1500 mg recommended in the United States. At levels of 250 to 400 mg of calcium per day, women in third world countries do not have the rates of osteoporosis and hip fractures common in developed countries. In addition, on the Fat Flush plan, all the "calcium robbers," such as caffeine, sugar, alcohol, and excess fiber from grains and bran, are totally eliminated, allowing you to retain all the calcium you consume.

However, if you still have concerns, you are welcome to experiment with other calcium-rich sources, such as sea vegetables or seaweeds. They are nutrition treasures from the deep, loaded with trace minerals in addition to the more common calcium and iron. For instance, you could try some hijiki. It tastes a lot like licorice and looks like tangled black strings, yet it has fourteen times the calcium of a glass of milk. You simply rinse it under cold water and soak it for approximately twenty minutes. Then you can toss it into your salad or Rose's Fat Flush Soup*! It also can be sautéed with carrots and fresh ginger.

FLUSH FLASH

Recipes for dishes marked with an asterisk can be found in Chapter 10.

Protein is an essential part of the Fat Flush Plan, but how much do I really need?

In the past, 1 gram of protein for every 2.2 pounds of body weight was the "gold standard." Now this has been changed as a result of new research suggesting that certain individuals may need much more: weight-lifters, individuals having a large, muscular frame, immunosuppressed individuals, and those suffering from protein deficiency (with such symptoms as prolonged water retention, sagging muscles, loss of muscle mass, expanding waistlines, fatigue, anemia, slow wound healing, hair thinning and loss). Practically doubling the previous recommendation, some authorities now recommend up to 1 to 1.5 grams of protein per pound of body weight.

So as far as exact amounts are concerned, the jury is still out. For years I have concurred with the Food and Nutrition Board of the National Research Council, which recommends the following amounts of protein as a general rule of thumb:

Adult men	70 grams
Adult women	58 grams
Pregnant women	65 grams
Lactating women	75 grams
Girls, aged 13–15	62 grams
Girls, aged 16–20	58 grams
Boys, aged 13–15	75 grams
Boys, aged 16–20	85 grams

To me, these numbers represent the bare minimum requirements, not the amounts for optimal health. The best way to figure out what works for you is by trial and error. You can add a couple of ounces of protein to lunch and dinner or include some high-protein, lactose-free whey shakes for snacks with your daily fruit.

Here are some examples that will help you keep track of your protein grams:

1 egg = 7 grams

1 ounce of meat, fish, fowl, or cheese = 7 grams

1 or 2 scoops of whey powder = 20 grams

4 ounces of tofu = 7 grams

2 ounces of tempeh = 7 grams

I'm a vegan. Is there anything special I should do—and what about using beans for my protein portions?

To be quite honest, since animal proteins play such an important role in the Fat Flush Plan, vegans will be challenged to find equivalent sources that provide the quality of amino acids found only in meat, eggs, fish, and poultry. The five most critical amino acids lacking in most vegan diets, according to biochemist Don Tyson, who ran the Aatron Medical Services Laboratory in Torrance, California, for years, are lysine, methionine, carnitine, taurine, and tryptophan.

Taking a well-balanced amino acid supplement containing lysine, methionine, carnitine, and taurine (tryptophan is no longer on the market) with meals would be a good first step. There is also a protein powder available, made from peas, that would be appropriate for vegans because it is enhanced with the four amino acids. Vegetarians, of course, can increase the whey protein shakes during the day and include a balanced amino acid supplement (as described above).

As for the beans, they are a source of protein, but they also contain significant amounts of carbohydrates. For instance, 8 ounces of chickpeas contain a whopping 120 grams of carbohydrates. Thus, beans are really considered a carbohydrate.

In phase 3 of the plan, you can start to include these back in your Lifestyle eating routine in very small amounts. (They are not part of phase 1 or phase 2.)

Is it really okay to eat egg yolks? I always thought that they were a trigger for high cholesterol.

Yes, it is perfectly okay to have two whole eggs every day in each phase of the Fat Flush Plan. Eggs contain one of the highest-quality proteins available in any food. In fact, the egg yolk contains 45 percent of the egg's protein, along with many minerals and a good deal of the egg's vitamins. Omega-3–enriched eggs are also available, which provide nearly 200 mg of cholesterol-lowering omega-3s concentrated in the yolk. (Please see Chapter 9 for more information.) The yolk is also an excellent source of the infection-fighting vitamin A and contains a nutrient called *phosphatidylcholine*. As part of the substance known as *lecithin*, phosphatidylcholine actually prevents the oxidation of cholesterol, which protects both your liver and your arteries.

In fact, numerous studies have vindicated the maligned egg yolk. The most recent studies have shown that adults can enjoy at least two eggs a day without increasing their serum cholesterol level. Two substantial Harvard studies, published in April 1999 in the *Journal of the American Medical Association (JAMA)*, examined the egg consumption of approximately 40,000 men and 80,000 women over an eight- to fourteen-year period. After taking into consideration other dietary patterns and risk factors, the researchers found that folks who ate one egg a day or more were no more likely to develop heart disease or stroke than those who consumed one egg a week or less. Researchers at Harvard Medical School actually sanction up to seven eggs per week for optimal health.

Thus, when it comes to breakfast on the Fat Flush Plan, you can count on eggs—poached, hard-cooked, soft-boiled, or scrambled. They are absolutely delicious poached or scrambled in vegetable or chicken broth. And you can enjoy them with low-glycemic vegetables, such as onions, mushrooms, or peppers, along with our special thermogenic herbs and spices, such as a dash of cayenne.

What about eating organ meats such as liver for a protein source?

Absolutely. Organ meats, such as liver and sweetbreads, are highly nutritious. In fact, liver is high in B vitamins, iron, and DHA—that important fatty acid so critical for the brain and eyes. When I was a WIC nutritionist at Bellevue Hospital in New York City many years ago, I discovered that many women suffering from anemia could increase their iron levels only by adding 4 ounces of calf's liver twice a week to their menu plan. The iron pills made them constipated. I still believe that liver can greatly benefit women who are menstruating and slightly anemic. Of course, organic liver is preferred.

Why isn't pork on the food list?

If you've ever looked at pork under a microscope, you would understand why it is not on any phase of the Fat Flush Plan. The *Trichinella spiralis* organism, which causes trichinosis, is rampant in American pigs. And even though you can neutralize the organism through Dr. Parcells' special food bath soak, who wants to be eating dead parasites? Or let's say you are out and happen to eat undercooked pork, bacon, or ham; the encysted larvae can hatch in your intestines and migrate to your muscles, where they mimic at least fifty other illnesses characterized by a persistent flu-like feeling and severe muscle aches and pains. Need I say more?

Is sushi allowed on the Fat Flush Plan when I eat out?

No, I don't recommend it. Raw fish can carry parasites (such as tapeworms and microscopic invaders), even more exotic ones such as the anisakine larvae. As I write in my book, *Guess What Came to Dinner: Parasites and Your Health,* when these small worms are ingested from raw or undercooked fish, they penetrate the walls of the stomach or small intestine, causing severe inflammation and pain. The symptoms can mimic appendicitis, gastric ulcer, or even stomach cancer. Surgical removal of the worms is a familiar surgery in Japan, where raw fish is a dietary staple.

Take it from me, these uninvited guests at your dinner table not only can become embedded in your intestines but also are at the source of irritable bowel syndrome, diarrhea, constipation, immune problems, and even depression in many cases. Since the Fat Flush Plan is a weight loss program that also cleanses your system, the last thing you want to do is introduce to your body such unpleasant and immunosuppressive critters that can rob you of vitality.

I understand why sugar is out on the Fat Flush Plan, but is a sugar substitute such as aspartame really going to upset my weight loss goals that badly?

Not only is aspartame suspected of stimulating insulin release and therefore counterproductive to your weight loss goals, but it also can damage your health.

The mere taste of such a concentrated sweetener appears to set an instinctual insulin mechanism into place even though aspartame contains zero calories. A six-year study of 80,000 women shows that the higher the artificial sweetener consumption, the more likely the women were to pack on the pounds.

Aspartame, marketed under the Equal and Nutrasweet brand names, also has been shown to suppress production of serotonin—the remarkable neurotransmitter that helps control food cravings. When serotonin levels plummet, those sugar and carb cravings skyrocket. And this increases the likelihood of binging and added pounds.

Loading up on those diet drinks—sweetened by aspartame—can rob you of valuable chromium, a mineral needed for proper blood sugar function. Having an insufficient amount of chromium results in poor blood sugar regulation, which can lead to insulin resistance and increased carb intolerance.

Does that also go for Splenda and Sweet'n Low?

They may be better choices, but I am still on the fence regarding their safety. The only brand-name sweetener I recommend is Stevia Plus, found in health food stores. Stevia is an herb used for hundreds of years in South America by Indian tribes in Paraguay. It is thirty times sweeter than regular sugar, is virtually calorie-free, and does not feed yeast, nor does it trigger fat-conserving insulin production or raise blood sugar levels like other sweeteners.

In terms of overall health, this natural herb is an antiflatulent and reduces heartburn, hypertension, and uric acid. Even researchers have gotten on the stevia bandwagon. A study in the *Journal of Ethnopharmacology* demonstrates how stevia dilates vessels, resulting in lower blood pressure and increased urine flow.

The Stevia Plus brand, unlike other stevias on the market, contains no added maltodextrin—an extremely high-glycemic substance. Instead, the natural sweetness of Stevia Plus is enhanced with fructooligosaccharides (FOSs), substances from natural grains and vegetables that provide a benefit that none of the other sweeteners do: It nourishes the growth of friendly bacteria, which are your best allies in keeping yeast such as *Candida* at bay. Remember that yeast overgrowth can make you want to overeat (see Chapter 2).

Is it all right to drink a vegetable juice such as V-8 on the Fat Flush Plan?

Yes, in phase 3, you can start drinking your veggies. However, please use only the low-sodium brands, such as Knudsen's, available at health food stores.

Are cooking sprays allowed?

Yes, but only in phase 3, the Lifestyle Eating Plan. And then, please use such sprays as olive oil cooking sprays only sparingly.

What about eating olives on the Fat Flush Plan?

Yes, yes, yes. They are included in all three phases of the Fat Flush Plan because they are high in oleic acid, a healthy fat that aids blood sugar and keeps insulin levels low. How many? Eating 3–6 per day would be fine.

SUBSTITUTIONS

I don't really like the taste of flax. What about substituting flax oil capsules for the flaxseed oil?

Yes, you can certainly do that—with caution. Sometimes in the process of encapsulation the oil's quality can be compromised. You might want to first test its quality by piercing the capsule and tasting the oil. It should have a nutty flavor. A bitter taste with an almost stinging-like aftertaste signals rancidity.

On another note, the flaxseed oil is far more economical than the capsules. However, if you travel frequently, the capsules may be more convenient. Just be certain to purchase a good-quality product. It takes about 9 capsules of flaxseed oil to equal 1 tablespoon of the liquid oil. Just remember that with the required 2 tablespoons of flaxseed oil daily, you would be taking 18 pills each day, staggering them throughout the day, say, 6 per meal.

Can ground-up flaxseeds be used in place of flaxseed oil?

Yes, they can. Use 3 tablespoons of ground-up flaxseeds to 1 tablespoon of the flaxseed oil. In phases 1 and 2, flaxseed meal can be sprinkled over your vegetables, mixed in your salad, or used in your fruit smoothies. In phase 3, you can add it to cottage cheese or yogurt. But if you use flaxseeds instead of flaxseed oil, use psyllium in the Long Life Cocktail.

And by using ground-up flaxseeds as a substitute, you get an extra bonus of about 8 grams of additional fiber with your meals. Flaxseed is also higher in lignans than the oil. Lignans, which are 800 times more concentrated in whole flaxseed than in other plants, are well recognized for their antioxidant properties, phytoestrogen help in alleviating perimenopausal and menopausal discomforts, and breast cancer–fighting abilities. In fact, a study conducted at the Princess Margaret Hospital and the Toronto Hospital in Canada showed how as little as 2 tablespoons a day of ground flaxseed markedly slowed down tumor growth in women with breast cancer. The tagline "A muffin a day could keep breast cancer at bay" hit the newswires on December 7, 2000, after the research was presented at an international conference on breast cancer in San Antonio, Texas. Lignans are also a soluble fiber, which keeps blood sugar levels stable and lowers cholesterol.

What about taking fish oil in place of flaxseed oil?

If you can't take flax for any reason, using a pharmaceutical-grade fish oil that has the PCBs and heavy metals removed is certainly a viable substitute. Because of fish oil's concentration, you would use 1 teaspoon of fish oil to 1 tablespoon of flaxseed oil. Because of the taste, you might want to add this to your morning smoothie, getting it all in one shot.

Both flaxseed and fish oils are the richest sources of the omega-3 fatty acids. In clinical studies, they have been found to burn nearly three times faster than animal fats. No wonder they are known as the "antiobesity fats."

Also, fish oils containing the omega-3 fatty acids EPA and DHA are linked to a variety of health-protective benefits. A number of studies have shown how fish oils promote a normal heart rhythm, prevent clots, increase circulation, inhibit inflammation, and lower triglycerides and blood pressure. In October 2000, the American Heart Association recommended that everyone eat at least two 3-ounce servings of fatty fish per week. Even the FDA has cautiously given the omega-3s its stamp of approval. In November 2000, the FDA announced: "The scientific evidence that omega-3s may reduce the risk of heart disease is suggestive."

The noted diet guru of *The Zone* fame, Barry Sears, Ph.D., believes that high-quality fish oil is the treatment of choice for neurologic disorders such as depression, ADHD, Alzheimer's disease, and Parkinson's disease. I recommend the liquid fish oil manufactured by the Sears Lab, Omega Rx (see Chapter 12).

May I substitute olive oil for flaxseed oil?

Sorry, no. Even though olive oil is a "heart smart," tasty oil that's great for cooking and part of the Lifestyle Eating Plan, it is not a substitute for flaxseed oil. Olive oil does not contain the essential fatty acids found in flax. Flaxseed oil not only possesses unique fat-burning power but also improves immune function, protects against heart disease, and improves male fertility. Fat Flushers who faithfully adopt the flax habit consistently remark about having glowing skin, luster-rich hair, and strong nails.

I can't find natural cranberry juice in my area. May I substitute another juice, or what would you suggest?

Please don't substitute another juice, because it negates the entire purpose of cranberry juice in the Fat Flush Plan. Cranberry juice is packed with flavonoids, enzymes, and organic acids, such as malic acid, citric acid, and quinic acid, which have an emulsifying effect on stubborn fat deposits in the lymphatic system. The lymphatic system, which has been called the "garbage collector of the body," transports all kinds of waste products not processed by the liver. With the help of the organic acid components, the cranberry juice digests stagnated lymphatic wastes, which could very well be the reason Fat Flushers claim that their cellulite disappears.

Here's what I suggest. If you can't find natural cranberry juice, there is a really simple recipe in Chapter 4 that you can use to make your own. Since it is pretty hard to find cranberries during nonholiday times, you might want to stock up when they're easily available in November and December and freeze them for future use.

I'm concerned about the carb content in the cranberry juice. What about taking concentrated cranberry capsules instead?

Concentrated cranberry capsules may be a great help in preventing or treating urinary tract infections. However, from my experience, there is no substitute for the unsweetened cranberry juice used in the cranberry juice–water mixture in phase 1 and in the more concentrated form in phases 2 and 3 with the Long Life Cocktail. Because it is liquid, the cranberry juice is absorbed immediately into the system, helping to keep the liver's detoxification pathways open and acting as a digestive aid for the waste material stuck in the lymphatic system.

The capsules can be difficult to digest for people who have inadequate stomach acid production or insufficient digestive enzymes. If you are concerned about the carbohydrate content of the unsweetened cranberry juice, don't be. The cranberry seems to act more as a catalyst for digesting stagnated lymphatic wastes than as a food source. There are approximately 15 grams of carbohydrate in 8 ounces—the daily amount called for in the Fat Flush Plan. And since it is being diluted with water, you are not consuming it all at once to overwhelm your system.

Is it all right if I substitute psyllium pills for the psyllium in the Long Life Cocktail?

Yes, you can substitute psyllium pills or other high-fiber supplements. Just be sure to follow the instructions on the label. Many Fat Flushers have used a product called Super GI Cleanse with much success. It's a well-balanced product that contains both soluble and insoluble fibers from psyllium, flax, oat bran, and pectin. The Super GI Cleanse targets the colon, liver, kidneys, lungs, and lymphatics with additional probiotics ("friendly bacteria") that compete with *Candida* and help keep yeast under control (see Chapter 12).

I can't take psyllium in any form. Is there a substitute?

Yes, there sure is. Take 1 tablespoon of ground flaxseeds in place of 1 teaspoon of psyllium.

You recommend whey protein, but can I use soy protein powders instead?

No. Although I allow soy products in the form of tofu and tempeh up to twice a week for the sake of the vegetarians and vegans who are on the Fat Flush Plan, I decided long ago that less is more when it comes to soy protein powders.

For starters, soy is not a complete protein because it lacks methionine, an important sulfur-bearing amino acid for liver detoxification. Soy is also a top food allergen and contains enzyme inhibitors and phytic acid, which can remove zinc and iron from the body. As a plentiful source of copper, soy can increase or exacerbate hyperactivity, panic attacks, hair loss, adrenal burnout, fatigue, and hypothyroidism. (For more information, please refer to my book, *Why Am I Always So Tired?*)

Whey protein is a much better protein powder choice. It has the highest protein efficiency ratio of all the protein sources and increases production of glutathione, one of the liver's leading antioxidants in the detox process.

I do think, however, that there is a place for soy isoflavones as a natural hormone-replacement therapy for perimenopausal and menopausal women (women in their early forties through middle fifties). In amounts up to 100 mg per day—the amounts Asians typically ingest on a daily basis—soy can be good medicine.

Can lime be substituted for lemon?

Certainly. You can substitute lime or mix the two, using half lemon and half lime.

SUPPLEMENTS AND MEDICATIONS

Do I have to take supplements while on the Fat Flush Plan?

You bet. Certain supplements—such as the essential fatty acids from GLA and flax as well as conjugated linoleic acid (CLA)—are really crucial to the success of the plan. These essential and critical fats are suggested throughout each phase for a specific purpose, with your weight and fat loss goals always in mind. The daily dose of 360 to 400 mg of GLA in the form of evening primrose, borage, or black currant seed oil helps trigger fat burning (instead of fat storage) by mobilizing brown adipose tissue (BAT), which burns off extra calories and increases energy. GLA also controls PMS symptoms and wards off rheumatoid arthritis and skin problems, such as psoriasis and eczema.

Research has proven that the one major obstacle to dieting is hunger. Taking 2 tablespoons daily of flaxseed oil eliminates this problem because it creates a feeling of fullness (satiety) and makes you feel fuller longer. You are happy with less food because you are less hungry. Flaxseed oil does this by revving up metabolism and eliminating the deprivation that can make you give in to temptation and cheat on your diet. In addition, the flaxseeds themselves are a powerful source of antioxidants and plant sterols, responsible for a major portion of human immune function.

In phase 3, you'll add 1000 mg of CLA before each meal, which will help your body burn fat even more. CLA is your fat-proof insurance policy. Even if you somehow regain some weight, you'll redeposit that weight as 50 percent muscle. And CLA even aids in the prevention of breast cancer by acting as a powerful antioxidant in the system. It doesn't get any better than this!

What other supplements can I take on the Fat Flush Plan?

A broad-based multivitamin and mineral supplement would be helpful as insurance. You also could add a weight loss formula that supports liver cleansing as well as carbohydrate and fat metabolism (see Chapter 12). Whatever brand you choose, the most important ingredients in a weight loss or fat-burning product are liver-protecting milk thistle and dandelion, blood sugar/insulin–controlling chromium, and methionine, inositol, choline, and L-carnitine for mobilizing fat. You are welcome to supplement your diet with formulas containing at least two to three of these ingredients.

There is, however, one other supplement that I would suggest—magnesium. Magnesium is particularly helpful on the Fat Flush Plan with those occasional headaches from caffeine withdrawal as well as challenges with constipation. Since magnesium is a major muscle relaxant, it helps restore good bowel tone and normal peristalsis—that alternating muscle relaxation and contraction in the intestines. Magnesium also helps the liver do its job more efficiently by acting as an escort for toxins being moved through the liver, including estrogens (such as those in the pill or HRT) being broken down. In addition, magnesium is key to good bone health, balancing calcium and converting vitamin D for better calcium absorption.

Magnesium deficiency is common in our twenty-first-century lifestyle, thanks to highly processed foods, birth control pills, and stress. Even though the recommended daily allowance (RDA) is 400 mg daily, most of us consume less than 100 mg. And those drinks many of us may have enjoyed BFF (Before Fat Flush!)—such as coffee, tea, alcohol, and colas—don't help. They wash magnesium right out of the system via the urine. Symptoms of a magnesium deficiency include nervousness, irritability, depression, fatigue, palpitations, tremors, and spasms. According to a 1990 study by Guy Abraham, M.D., a magnesium deficiency also will reduce blood calcium, which decreases calcium availability for your bones and further disrupts estrogen metabolism.

I would suggest taking magnesium separately from calcium, because it needs to be absorbed by itself. You can take from 400 to 1200 mg daily, depending on bowel tolerance. You can build up to these amounts slowly if you notice any bowel intolerance.

Does the Pill interact with the psyllium husks in the Long Life Cocktail?

Yes. The water-soluble fiber in the psyllium can inhibit the effectiveness of birth control pills and any other prescription medications (including desiccated thyroid). Therefore, you shouldn't take them at the same time you drink the Long Life Cocktail. Instead, take your medications several hours before or after the cocktail.

Since I started on Depo-Provera, I've gained a lot of weight. What do you suggest?

Get off of Depo-Provera and find an alternative method as soon as you can! Depo-Provera, that injectable form of progestin frequently used for birth control, can cause your body to hold onto more fluid. The concentrated progestins are the culprits. They decrease insulin sensitivity, which can add even more fat to the water weight.

There are many low-dose birth control pills on the market. However, as discussed in Chapter 2, all synthetic hormones—including those from birth control pills—put undue stress on the liver and can back up the detoxification pathways. Ultimately, this impairs bile flow, which will affect your ability to burn fat. It is no wonder that women can gain up to 30 pounds while using Depo-Provera.

If you do get off of Depo-Provera and onto another method, I also would encourage you to fortify your liver and enhance its ability to break down estrogens and progestins. Many of these liver-supporting nutrients are included in the Fat Flush supporting nutrients described throughout the book. You can add more of them in the following amounts for even better liver fortification:

✓ MILK THISTLE: A powerful antioxidant that protects your liver from cell damage. It also is considered a liver regenerator and helps with bile stagnation. Take 500 to 2000 mg daily.
✓ DANDELION: Used for centuries worldwide as a liver tonic and blood purifier. Take 500 to 2000 mg daily.
✓ GLOBE ARTICHOKE: Another excellent blood purifier, also shown to lower blood cholesterol and help restore a damaged liver. Take 300 to 500 mg daily.

I'm on Prozac—but want to get off after reading how these kinds of antidepressants interfere with weight loss. Any suggestions?

Yes indeed. And by the way, you are not alone battling depression—nearly 20 million Americans suffer from it. If you are getting off of Prozac or any similar medications (such as Zoloft), you must do this under the care of a physician. Then you may want to investigate a breakthrough product called Ultra H-3, which balances the levels of the enzyme monoamine oxidase (MAO) in the brain. If MAO builds up in the brain, it replaces other vital substances such as norepinephrine (a hormone essential to well-being and vitality) and can cause depression as well as premature aging.

Based on over 500 laboratory studies of the legendary Romanian Ultra H-3 product, Ultra H-3 is a safe and effective remedy for depression when taken for a trial period of at least three months (see Chapter 12).

Should I avoid over-the-counter products such as ibuprofen or cold medicines while on the Fat Flush Plan? What about taking Celexa, Prevacid, Claritin, or the diet drug Xenical—or even antibiotics—while on the Fat Flush Plan?

It is best to avoid over-the-counter medicines and prescription drugs while on the Fat Flush Plan, because they all need to be broken down by the liver. One of the main purposes of the Fat Flush Plan is to protect your primary fat-burning organ, the liver, through cleansing and gentle detoxification. Increasing its workload at this time wouldn't be advisable.

You need to be especially cautious with Tylenol, which has been found to be toxic to liver function.

Keep in mind also that if you come down with a cold when your sinuses start to act up or if you start to have digestive problems, these could simply be symptoms of your cleansing process. And this is a good thing, because it means that the plan is working and you're on the way to your weight loss goals. Usually, these detoxification symptoms disappear in about four days.

If you happen to become ill while on the Fat Flush plan and you are sure it's not related to the cleansing process—such as a sore throat, the flu, or anything similar that requires medical attention—stop the plan and consult your physician. This is not the best time for you to do the Fat Flush Plan. Wait until you are well, and then begin again.

Are there any drug-nutrient interactions I should be aware of while following the Fat Flush Plan?

Yes, there are. The most important drug-nutrient interactions you should be aware of are as follows:

- ✓ **EVENING PRIMROSE OIL:** You shouldn't take antidepressants (such as Wellbutrin) with evening primrose oil, because it can augment the risk of seizures. This also holds true for individuals having psychotic disorders or taking phenothiazine drugs such as Thorazine, Mellaril, or Stelazine.
- ✓ **BORAGE OIL:** This has been shown to increase the blood-thinning qualities of medications such as aspirin, Dalteparin, Enoxaparin, and warfarin.
- ✓ **PSYLLIUM:** Taking psyllium with certain medications, such as Coumadin (an anticoagulant), Lanoxin (a heart medication), Tegretol (a seizure medication), or lithium (for manic depression) is not advised. Also remember that fiber can inhibit the pills' effectiveness. So stagger the meals with your Long Life Cocktail.

EXERCISE

I am an exercise freak. Do I have to change my routine while on the Fat Flush Plan?

Yes, it would be best for the first two phases. Since the Fat Flush plan also cleanses your system as it helps you drop those extra pounds, stick with low to moderate exercises, such as those suggested in Chapter 7, while on the first two phases. You'll find the brisk walking for thirty minutes and a minitrampoline workout will help keep released toxins moving out of the lymphatic system and out of the body. Later on, you may add more intense weight-bearing exercises when you reach phase 3 of the program.

I hate to exercise—even if it's just walking. Do I have to?

Absolutely—for the best results. As I stated earlier, the exercises on the Fat Flush Plan are easy but necessary to escort toxins out of your body and to protect your lymphatic health. And besides, you just might enjoy it. I find my power walks inspiring. They release tension and free my mind. And that in itself helps reduce stress and those urges to binge. In addition, walking conditions the heart and respiratory system, pumping oxygen to all parts of the body. It even helps your body's response to insulin (another hidden weight gain factor).

Why not grab a friend or family member? The minutes will fly by, and you'll get in some good quality time to boot. Or you can don some headphones and listen to your favorite tunes.

COFFEE, TEA, OR . . . ?

May I at least have one cup of coffee a day?

If this is what it will take to keep you on the Fat Flush Plan, then go ahead and have just one cup of coffee a day. Just make certain that you thoroughly read Chapter 3 so that you are aware that over 200 pesticides are used on many coffee plants and that regular coffee (as well as decaf) is the most toxic substance for your liver to metabolize. Similar to the insulin effect from aspartame, caffeine can block your weight loss efforts. And I'm not just talking about the caffeine in coffee—this also goes for black tea, green tea, iced tea, dark or milk chocolate, colas, and over-the-counter drugs such as cold medicines, pain relievers, and allergy remedies.

And keep in mind, if you will, that coffee is a heavy-duty diuretic that strips calcium, magnesium, and sodium from your body—the very minerals you need for bone building. In fact, caffeine from coffee, tea, and soft drinks doubles the rate of calcium excretion. Three cups of black coffee can results in a 45-mg calcium loss. Thus, it is no wonder that a six-year study conducted by the Department of Medicine at Boston's Brigham and Women's Hospital in the early 1980s showed a remarkable connection between caffeine and hip fractures. The researchers tracked 84,484 women from the ages of 34 to 59. Interestingly, the women who experienced a three times higher risk of hip fractures also had a higher intake of caffeine.

I was an avid coffee drinker and finally switched to green tea. Do I really have to give that up as well?

All I can say is this: Caffeine is caffeine is caffeine. Although green tea contains about a third of the caffeine of a drip-brewed cup of regular coffee—35 mg in green tea and 100 mg in regular coffee per 6 ounces to be exact—even this lesser amount can overload the liver and inhibit its fat-burning duties. This is especially true if you are already taking birth control pills or HRT, which are very hard on the liver already. Thus, you would be adding insult to injury.

Also, both black tea and green tea are naturally high in copper, a mineral potentially overabundant in many unsuspecting women. Excess copper can impair the conversion of thyroid hormones, resulting in hypothyroidism. And when this occurs, your energy production slows down, you feel tired, and your weight can escalate.

In phase 3 you can enjoy no-caffeine herbal teas to your heart's content. Until then, it's water to the rescue or even more hot water with lemon while you're in phases 1 and 2.

What about alcohol—is it okay on the weekend or a special occasion?

Once you graduate to phase 3, the Lifestyle Eating Plan, anything in moderation is fine. However, during phases 1 and 2, when we are trying to give the liver a well-deserved vacation, I really prefer that you abstain. When you drink alcohol in any form, it not only drains magnesium but also becomes the fuel of choice for your body to burn. And if your body is busy processing alcohol, it can't burn stored fat—and this inhibits the fat-burning process altogether. In addition, alcohol feeds yeast. Yeast-related toxins are extremely disruptive to your liver (the body's premier fat-burning organ) and serve to practically shut down the fat-burning process.

OTHER CONCERNS

What if I slip and chow down a hefty pasta meal with all the trimmings—am I doomed to gaining all my weight back?

No, you are just human, like all of us. Although one meal won't put your weight back on, you'll probably not feel too terrific afterward. In fact, you'll more than likely feel tired or bloated. This will be enough of an incentive to help you stay more on track. And remember that the beauty of the Fat Flush Plan is that you can jump back to phase 1 whenever you get off base—like after a major holiday celebration.

It's my third day on the Fat Flush plan, and I have a caffeine withdrawal headache and am very tired. Is this normal?

Yes, it is a normal reaction to cleansing and the withdrawal from coffee as well as sugar, grains, and dairy foods—especially if you've been a big consumer of these items. According to nutritional biochemist Stephen Cherniske, M.S.:

> A caffeine deprivation (withdrawal) headache results from the normal opening (dilation) of blood vessels that are constricted by caffeine. In other words, habitual caffeine intake keeps blood vessels in the brain constricted. When caffeine is not consumed, these blood vessels return to their normal blood flow potential, and it is this increased circulation in the brain that causes the throbbing

agony of a caffeine withdrawal headache. Ultimately, the brain becomes accustomed to normal blood flow and the headache subsides. And the caffeine headache connection goes well beyond withdrawal. Caffeine itself contributes to headache even when it is consumed moderately and consistently.

Don't fret. After the first four days, you'll find many of your symptoms vanishing, especially the headaches—if you take it easy, rest, and follow the exercise advice outlined in Chapter 7.

I'm in phase 2—the transition part of the Fat Flush Plan—and seem to have reached a plateau. What should I do?

For starters, you need to know that you're not technically on a plateau unless you've stopped dropping weight for at least three weeks. And reaching a plateau is common, regardless of the weight plan you're following.

Since phase 2 adds two portions of the friendly carbs back into the menu, you may want to look a bit closer at this issue. Are you following the plan as suggested, or have you inadvertently overshot the carb allowances? You also may want to cut back on recipes containing onions or tomatoes, which are higher-carb veggies. Although healthful, cleansing foods, they can be a hidden source of weight-gaining carbs for some people. For instance, ½ cup of onions has 7.4 g of carbohydrates, and a medium-size raw tomato (2½ inch) has 5.8 g, 1 cup of canned tomatoes has 10 g, and 1 cup of tomato juice has 10.4 g.

Here's where the beauty of the Fat Flush Plan can come into play. You can go back to phase 1 for a week, cutting back on all carbs to see how you do. If this causes you to lose weight, then watching your carb levels from here on out is your primary concern. So be on the lookout for hidden sugars, and read labels.

To help you achieve this, I would greatly recommend sticking to the journaling ritual. It will provide you with a clear picture of what and how much you are consuming—and reveal if there are any other ways you may be secretly sabotaging your weight loss.

You also may want to add CLA to your regimen, which is really part of phase 3. As you may remember from my discussion in Chapter 2, research over the past twenty years has shown that CLA reduces the body's ability to store fat for energy by controlling the enzymes that release fat from the cells into the bloodstream. The result is a decrease in body fat and a proportional increase in lean muscle mass.

Organic foods can get pricey—especially on my limited budget. What can I do?

Many years ago, my mentor, Dr. Hazel Parcells, discovered an economical yet highly effective way to remove pesticides, bacteria, parasites, and other contaminants from food. I have been using this special food soak for over twenty years and describe it in Chapter 9. You can use it to cleanse leafy, root, and thick-skinned veggies, as well as thin or thick-skinned fruits and poultry, fish, meat, and eggs

I'm having a problem with constipation on the diet. What should I do?

I would check to make sure that you are adding enough water. You may also want to add 400 mg of magnesium in the morning and 400 mg in the evening, because this helps to relax the intestinal walls and establish normal peristalsis.

Should I be watching my stools during the Fat Flush Plan, and what am I looking for exactly?

Believe it or not, your stools reveal telltale signs of what's going on with your body. Here are four areas to watch for:

- ✓ SMELL: No, they really don't have to have a foul odor. But if they do, it's a sign that putrefaction—rotting and fermentation of food—is occurring in your digestive tract. This means that your bad bacteria are more than likely outweighing your friendly bacteria. And this spells trouble, because it's your good bacteria that help digest food by creating digestive enzymes and keeping the bad bacteria under control.
- ✓ FREQUENCY: Actually, having two to three bowel movements a day is considered healthy. You want to keep things moving along so that stagnation and putrefaction don't occur. This is where the fiber (psyllium or ground flaxseeds) comes into play to help you eliminate more readily and thereby ward off disease.
- ✓ FORMATION: Generally speaking, a 2-foot-long stool with a diameter about the size of a half dollar is considered the best. Anything short of this could mean that you're lacking fiber, flora, or the enzymes needed to ensure complete digestion. If food particles (notably protein) are not broken down completely, they can enter the bloodstream, which leads the way to food allergies, a weakened immune system, and various diseases.
- ✓ FLOTATION: If your stools sink to the bottom of the toilet, it means that they are too hard and that your diet is lacking something, possibly fiber and/or essential fatty acids. A healthy stool floats, is not compact, and breaks into smaller pieces as it is flushed.

Will I ever be able to have my favorite white flour foods again, such as pasta, white bread, and other carbohydrates?

Of course you can. By the time you are ready for these white flour favorites, however, I hope that you will have lost your taste for them and balanced your body chemistry so that you can enjoy them in moderation, for example, a half a cup here and there and on special occasions.

I hope you'll crave the friendly carbs instead, such as whole-grain sprouted breads, peas, carrots, and even sweet potatoes and squash. When I am in the mood for more carbs, I slice up a squash, spread the slices on a baking sheet, and bake it in a 325°F oven for thirty minutes. I make believe that I am having french fries. The slices are quite delicious with some cinnamon or cloves.

Can I ever have popcorn again?

Yes, you can have all your favorite foods. Once you graduate to phase 3 and add back friendly carbs, you might even consider drizzling 1 tablespoon of flaxseed oil on your popcorn, the way I do.

CHAPTER

12 Resources

Good information is your best medicine.

—MICHAEL E. DEBAKEY, M.D.

If you would like to read the most inspiring testimonials, find out which products have the Fat Flush seal of approval, and learn about all the latest nutritional buzz in the media, visit my Web site. This site also will present you with information on how to keep up with me and my schedule: *www.annlouise.com.*

FAT FLUSH RESOURCES

As a convenience for my readers and clients, Uni Key Health Systems has been the main distributor of my products, books, and services over the years. Uni Key carries the Fat Flush Kit (see below), high-lignan flaxseed oil and flaxseed oil capsules, CLA 1000, Ultra H-3, Super GI Cleanse, Y-C Cleanse, Progesta-Key natural topical progesterone cream, the Doulton Water Filter Systems, and Royal Prestige Cookware; it also provides services for salivary hormone testing. You may call for a catalog of the latest products and also order all my books through them.

Uni Key Health Systems
P.O. Box 7168
Bozeman, MT 59771
1-800-888-4353
www.unikeyhealth.com
unikey@unikeyhealth.com

The Fat Flush Kit

The Fat Flush Kit, in conjunction with the Fat Flush Plan diet, can be an effective way to lose fat, banish cellulite, lose inches, and tone your body. Free of harsh stimulants such as ephedra (ma huang), caffeine, and aspirin, the kit consists of a gamma-linolenic acid (GLA) supplement, a weight loss formula, and a dieter's multivitamin. These three products safely help to ensure proper nutrient intake during weight loss, reestablish a beneficial fat ratio in the brown fat tissues for continued weight stabilization, trigger fat burning (thermogenesis), aid in appetite control, suppress cravings, and support and nourish our tired and overworked livers.

GLA-90 (Cold-Pressed Black Currant Seed Oil)

120 softgels

Each capsule contains 100 percent black currant seed oil, providing 90 mg of GLA.

Weight Loss Formula

90 capsules

Three capsules contain vitamin B_3, 15 mg; vitamin B_6, 20 mg; vitamin C, 100 mg; choline, 335 mg; inositol, 200 mg; chromium, 400 mcg; L-lysine hydrochloride, 100 mg; D,L-methionine, 335 mg; L-carnitine tartrate, 500 mg; soya lecithin, 100 mg; lipase plant enzyme, 200 mg; and lipotropic herbal blend (turmeric, dandelion root, milk thistle, Oregon graperoot), 200 mg.

Dieter's Multivitamin and Minerals (Iodine- and Iron-Free)

60 Capsules

Two capsules contain vitamin A (beta-carotene), 10,000 IU (International Units); vitamin C, 180 mg; vitamin D, 800 IU; vitamin E, 60 IU; vitamin B_1, 6 mg; vitamin B_2, 6.8 mg; vitamin B_3, 60 mg; vitamin B_5, 20 mg; vitamin B_6, 6 mg; vitamin B_{12},18 mg; folic acid, 800 mg; biotin, 600 mg; calcium, 120 mg; magnesium, 200 mg; potassium, 15 mg; phosphorus, 92 mg; zinc, 30 mg; copper, 2 mg; manganese, 8 mg; chromium, 200 mcg; selenium, 200 mcg; and molybdenum, 100 mcg.

OTHER NAME-BRAND NATURAL WEIGHT LOSS PRODUCTS

Individual Fat-Burning Nutrients

Many of these health food products are available in your local health food store, online, or through The Vitamin Shoppe (800-223-1216), which provides up to 30 percent discounts.

GLA

The Vitamin Shoppe Evening Primrose Oil, 500 mg (GLA, 45 mg)

Country Life Evening Primrose Oil, 500 mg (GLA, 45 mg)

Solaray Evening Primrose Oil, 500 mg (GLA, 50 mg)

Carlson's Evening Primrose Oil, 500 mg (GLA, 45 mg)

Health from the Sun Evening Primrose Oil, 500 mg (GLA, 45 mg)

EPA/DHA

Omega Rx, 8.8 fluid ounces (www.drsears.com)

Chromium

The Vitamin Shoppe Chromium Complex, 200 mcg

Country Life Chromium Complex (chromate), 200 mcg

KAL Chromium Picolinate, 200 mcg

Natrol Chromium Picolinate, 200 mcg

Nature's Plus Chromax (chromium picolinate), 200 mcg

Choline/Inositol

The Vitamin Shoppe Choline and Inositol, 250 mg of each

Country Life Choline/Inositol, 500 mg of each

KAL Choline/Inositol, 500 mg each

Nature's Plus Choline, 600 mg

Nature's Plus Inositol, 600 mg

Carnitine

Douglas Labs L-Carnitine (with Vitamin B_6), 500 mg

Country Life L-Carnitine (with Vitamin B_6), 500 mg

GNC L-Carnitine, 500 mg

Twin Labs L-Carnitine, 500 mg

Natrol L-Carnitine, 500 mg

Optimum Nutrition Liquid L-Carnitine (with Vitamin B_6), 2 tablespoons provide 1000 mg

Conjugated Linoleic Acid (CLA)

Tonalin, CLA 1000 mg (Look for Tonalin CLA under such brand names as GNC, Vitamin World, Nature's Way, Jarrow Formulas, and Natrol.)

Lipotropic Herbs

Many companies sell liver-supporting and regenerating herbs, in either the standardized or the whole-herb form, from turmeric, dandelion root, milk thistle, and Oregon grape root. Many of these are sold in health food stores or can be reached through the following telephone numbers and Web sites:

Nature's Way, 1-801-489-1500
www.naturesway.com

Bioforce, 1-877-232-6060
www.bioforce.com

EDUCATIONAL RESOURCES

Nutritional Organizations

American Menopause Foundation
The Empire State Building
350 Fifth Avenue
Suite 2822
New York, NY 10118
1-212-714-2398

The American Menopause Foundation is the only independent, not-for-profit organization dedicated to providing support and assistance on all issues concerning the change of life. Marie Lugano, the director, is a dynamo. She is dedicated to educating the public about all aspects of female health. The foundation's newsletter, literature, and educational programs provide the latest information on scientific research and other pertinent facts.

Certification Board for Nutrition Specialists
300 S. Duncan Avenue, Suite 225
Clearwater, FL 33755
1-727-446-6086/7958 (voice)
1-727-446-6202 (fax)
office@cert-nutrition.org
www.cert-nutrition.org

The board was organized in 1993 by the American College of Nutrition to satisfy the need for a valid certification for advanced-degreed nutritionists. Rigorous requirements have been established, including an advanced degree in nutrition or a closely related subject from a regionally accredited institution, significant experience in the field, and successful performance on a carefully designed examination. The examination has been given more than ten times since 1995 and is given two to three times per year at various locations. Recertification is required at five-year intervals.

The Society of Certified Nutritionists
2111 Bridgeport Way West, No. 2
University Place, WA 98466
1-800-342-8037
www.certifiednutritionist.com

As a graduate of American Health Science University, a certified nutritionist is dedicated to analyzing and arranging nutritional programs designed to meet the client's needs. Areas of expertise include counseling, advising, coordinating, educating, and client support. Many opportunities are available to qualified nutritionists. Professional, associate, and student memberships as well as corporate sponsorships are available in the Society of Certified Nutritionists.

The Candida and Dysbiosis Information Foundation
P.O. Drawer JF
College Station, TX 77841-5146

The Candida and Dysbiosis Information Foundation (CDIF), formerly known as Candida Research and Information Foundation (CRIF), is a private, nonprofit health organization created for the purpose of public education and patient support services as well as for data collection on chronic illnesses suspected of having a fungal/mycotoxic etiology. A special emphasis is given to conditions that are characterized by an imbalanced intestinal microflora ecology (i.e., dysbiosis).

Price-Pottenger Nutrition Foundation
P.O. Box 2614
La Mesa, CA 91943-2614
1-619-462-7600

The Price-Pottenger Nutrition Foundation is a nonprofit, tax-exempt educational organization dedicated to the promotion of enhanced health through awareness of ecology, lifestyle, and health food production and sound nutrition. At its core are the landmark works of Drs. Weston A. Price and Francis M. Pottenger, Jr., pioneers in modern research.

The American College for Advancement in Medicine (ACAM)
23121 Verdug Drive
Suite 204
Laguna Hills, CA 92653
1-800-532-3688

For a referral to a medical doctor or osteopath who is knowledgeable about alternative medicine and the use of natural hormone replacement, you can contact the ACAM.

The American Association of Naturopathic Physicians
2366 East Lake Avenue
Suite 322
Seattle, WA 98102

For a referral to a naturopathic physician who can guide you with natural hormone therapy, you can contact the American Association of Naturopathic Physicians.

Medical Nutrition Centers and Laboratories

The Health Research Institute and Pfeiffer Treatment Center
1804 Centre Point Circle
Naperville, IL 60563
1-630-505-0300

The Pfeiffer Treatment Center is a nonprofit medical research and treatment facility in Naperville, Illinois, specializing in research and treatment of biochemical imbalances. Since the center opened in 1989, it has treated more than 9000 patients who suffer from behavioral dysfunctions, depression, schizophrenia, bipolar disorder, autism, learning disorders, or anxiety by balancing body and brain chemistry. Pfeiffer's newest program focus is on natural, clinical approaches to the biochemical aspects of life-cycle changes of both men and women, such as aging, menopause, and puberty. The Pfeiffer Treatment Center, a branch of the Health Research Institute (HRI), is staffed by a team of physicians, chemists, and other professionals specializing in the effects of biochemistry on behavior, thought, or mood. The on-site HRI pharmacy compounds nutrients, hormones, and other biochemicals to reduce the number of pills in a prescription using customized methods and equipment.

MetaMetrix Clinical Laboratory
5000 Peachtree Industrial Blvd.
Norcross, GA 30071
1-800-221-4640
www.metametrix.com

MetaMetrix provides state-of-the-art blood tests and urine tests that detect underlying patterns of health. The laboratory also has specialty tests that detect fatty acid imbalances, which relate to degenerative diseases. The laboratory provides the only quantitative analysis of fatty acids available. This has been very useful in the prevention and treatment of heart disease, reproductive disorders, skin disorders, cancer, inflammatory bowel syndrome, arthritis, and childhood development disorders.

Magazines and Newsletters

The Woman's Health Letter
P.O. Box 467939
Atlanta, GA 31146-7939
1-800-728-2288

Nan Kathryn Fuchs, Ph.D., is the editor-in-chief and most definitely my kind of nutritionist. Her comments regarding health, nutrition, and medicine as they relate to women are timely and based on years of experience. I highly recommend that you consider subscribing to this fine health letter.

Health Sciences Institute
105 West Monument Street
Baltimore, MD 21201
1-800-981-7157

As a member of the professional advisory panel, I can verify that this cutting-edge newsletter is devoted to presenting extraordinary products to its members before the products hit the marketplace. They were the first to break the Ultra H-3 story—the extraordinary product for arthritis, depression, and antiaging. The Health Sciences Institute provides private access to hidden cures, powerful discoveries, breakthrough treatments, and advances in modern underground medicine.

Mercola Newsletter
www.mercola.com

One of the most comprehensive and well-researched newsletters on the Net.

Nutrition News
4108 Watkins Drive
Riverside, CA 92507
1-909-784-7500 or 800-784-7550
www.nutritionnews.com

Siri Khalsa is a wonderful veteran journalist who has been in the business of providing health education for over twenty-five years. Her easy-to-read newsletter covers a wide variety of contemporary and current topics. It is distributed in health food stores throughout the country, but you can subscribe directly.

Totalhealth for Longevity
165 North 100 East, Suite 2
St. George, UT 84770-9963
1-800-788-7806
sgmth@infowest.com
www.totalhealthmagazine.com

I am an associate editor for *Totalhealth for Longevity*. It is a comprehensive voice in antiaging, longevity, and self-managed natural health. Lyle Hurd, publisher extraordinaire, strives to bring readers fresh new information and perspectives on all phases of longevity medicine so that you can make an educated decision on the quality of your life today—and tomorrow.

Taste for Life
86 Elm Street
Peterborough, NH 03458
1-603-924-9692
mredd@tasteforlife.com
www.tasteforlife.com

Taste for Life is one of the fastest-growing in-store magazines for health food stores, natural product chains, food co-ops, and supermarkets nationwide. Its excellent articles on pertinent health issues offer readers an informative educational source on a variety of levels. I am proud to sit on Taste for Life's editorial board.

The Felix Letter
P.O. Box 7094
Berkeley, CA 94707

Nutritionist Clara Felix provides a delightful newsletter with a special focus on oils, hormone replacement, and the latest fountains of youth. I just love her original illustrations and cartoons.

Dr. Jonathan V. Wright's Nutrition and Healing
Agora South, LLC
819 North Charles Street
Baltimore, MD 21201
1-800-851-7100

Nutrition and Healing is dedicated to helping you keep yourself and your family healthy by the safest and most effective means possible. Every month you'll get information about diet, vitamins, minerals, herbs, natural hormones, and other substances and techniques to prevent and heal illness while prolonging your healthy life span.

Women's Health Access Newsletter
Corporate Office
429 Gammon Place
P.O. Box 259690
Madison, WI 53723
1-800-558-7046

This national newsletter features the latest developments in self-help tips regarding women's health issues such as PMS, menopause, natural hormone-replacement therapy, antioxidants, and preventive care.

Let's Live
320 North Larchmont Blvd.
P.O. Box 74908
Los Angeles, CA 90004
1-310-445-7500
www.letsliveonline.com

Boasting the largest circulation of all magazines in the natural foods market, *Let's Live* is a monthly publication with cutting-edge articles about all facets of health and fitness.

Herbs for Health
243 East Fourth Street
Loveland, CO 80537
1-970-663-0831

Herbs for Health is devoted to presenting the latest herbal scientific updates, legislative issues, and the whole range of benefits of herbs, including their role in the various healing arts.

Books for Your Bookshelf

Here is a listing and brief descriptions of my books that are excellent companions for your Fat Flush journey.

Eat Fat, Lose Weight Cookbook
Ann Louise Gittleman, M.S., C.N.S.
ISBN 0-658-01220-7
McGraw-Hill, 1999

The *Eat Fat, Lose Weight Cookbook* helps you say farewell to the cuisine of deprivation and introduces you to a whole new cuisine of celebration. With over 150 original recipes and a twenty-one-day sample plan using the amazing omega-3 "fat burning" fats from fish, flax, nuts, seeds, and avocados, you will lose weight and feel great. Good for the kids and the whole family—and they'll never know these enticingly delicious foods are healthy for them, too.

Eat Fat, Lose Weight
Ann Louise Gittleman, M.S., C.N.S.
ISBN 0-87983-966-X
Keats Publishing, 1999

Fat is your best friend, not your enemy, when it comes to weight loss. Learn all about the omega-3 fats—including fish, flax, olive oil, avocado, and evening primrose oil and borage oil—and how these friendly fats can burn excess body fat, lower cholesterol, heal depression, and increase your energy and alertness. Do check out the special "Fat Zappers" section.

The Living Beauty Detox Program
Ann Louise Gittleman, M.S., C.N.S.
ISBN 0-06251-628-0
HarperSanFrancisco, 2000

My Living Beauty Detox Program helps women of all ages determine their seasonal type using specially designed quizzes and offers regimens to resolve the problems that can plague women of every beauty type. Here you will find the beauty fundamentals every woman needs to maintain a healthier, more radiant appearance. Check out my favorite chapter, "Beauty Routines for Ages and Stages."

Beyond Pritikin
Ann Louise Gittleman, M.S., C.N.S.
ISBN 0-553-57400-0
Bantam Books, 1988

This is where it all began! My first book introduced the world to my Two-Week Fat Flush, which then became excerpted on iVillage.com, which received hundreds of thousands of hits per month. As the first nutritionist in the country to witness the pluses and minuses of a fat-free diet, I tell you everything you always wanted to know about curbing those crazy carbohydrates, fats, cholesterol, triglycerides, and fat-burning nutrients.

Why Am I Always So Tired?
Ann Louise Gittleman, M.S., C.N.S.
ISBN 0-06251-569-1
HarperSan Francisco, 1999

This book presents a groundbreaking discovery on the overlooked connection between exhaustion and a copper/zinc imbalance in our bodies. You will be amazed to read about the copper connection to other disorders such as hyperactivity, panic attacks, depression, skin conditions, and hormonal imbalances. Copper is found in water pipes, IUDs, and birth control pills (estrogen stockpiles copper) as well as in soy products, chocolate, and regular tea.

Before the Change
Ann Louise Gittleman, M.S., C.N.S.
ISBN 0-06-2515367-3
HarperSan Francisco, 1998

Before the Change offers the first complete do-it-yourself program for managing perimenopause—the period of about ten years leading up to menopause—with proven techniques for understanding and controlling its symptoms without powerful drugs or hormone treatments. The "Peri Zappers" that have been created in the book have changed women's lives immensely. Just take a look at the testimonials on amazon.com and see what I mean!

Guess What Came To Dinner
Parasites and Your Health (Revised and Updated)
Ann Louise Gittleman, M.S., C.N.S.
ISBN 1-58333-096-8
Avery, 2001

Parasites are alive and well in twenty-first century America. Learn how to protect yourself and your family from this alarming epidemic, which knows no economic or social boundaries. Parasites can masquerade as numerous illnesses, and this book masterfully covers everything you wanted to know and more about the warning signs, the water and food connection, man's best friend, diagnosis, treatment, and prevention.

Here are my personal all-time favorite related books:

The Ultimate Book of Women's Health
Nan Kathryn Fuchs, Ph.D.
ISBN 1-885385-01-3
Soundview Publications, Inc., 2001
1-800-728-2288

Dr. Fuchs gives us over 500 pages of proven ways to heal the female body.

Preventing and Reversing Osteoporosis
Alan R. Gaby, M.D.
ISBN 0-7615-0022-7
Prima Publishing, 1995

Dr. Gaby presents the best and most balanced view on osteoporosis that I have ever read.

Nutrition and Physical Degeneration
Weston Price, D.D.S.
ISBN: 0879838167
Keats Publishing, 1997

Nutrition and Physical Degeneration is one of the most important nutrition books ever written. Dr. Weston Price circled the globe in the early 1930s and made many striking discoveries about the danger of refined foods such as white flour and sugar and the benefits of meat and other animal products. It is one of the most complete reviews of what kinds of diets make people healthy.

The Age-Free Zone
Barry Sears, Ph.D.
ISBN 0-06098-832-0
Regan Books, 2000

In this breakthrough book, Dr. Sears goes beyond looking at food simply as a source of calories and explains the incredibly powerful biological effects it has on your hormones.

The Zone
Barry Sears, Ph.D.
ISBN 0-060391-150-2
HarperCollins, 1995

Barry Sears looks at why Americans are still overweight despite following the advice of experts.

Mastering the Zone
Barry Sears, Ph.D.
ISBN 0-060390190-1
Harper Collins, 1996

This book not only presents delicious, completely original *Zone*-favorable recipes that are easy to prepare and taste as good as they are good for you but also offers a practical guide to fine-tuning your *Zone* experience.

Mental and Elemental Nutrients: A Physician's Guide to Nutrition and Health Care
Carl C. Pfeiffer, Ph.D., M.D.
ISBN 0-87983-114-6
Keats Publishing, 1975

A classic book on the subject of mental and elemental nutrients.

Nutrition and Mental Illness: An Orthomolecular Approach to Balancing Body Chemistry
Carl C. Pfeiffer, Ph.D., M.D.
ISBN 0-89281-226-5
Inner Traditions International, Ltd, 1987

This book gives outstanding protocols regarding the orthomolecular way to treat mental illness.

The Healing Diet
G. M. Lemole, M.D.
ISBN 0-68817-073-0
William Morrow and Company, 2000

Dr. Lemole explains that by keeping the lymphatic system clear, we can eliminate 70 percent of chronic illnesses.

False Fat Diet
Elson Haas, M.D., and Cameron Stauth
ISBN 0-34544-315-2
Ballantine Books, 2001

A great title and a wonderfully written book that targets a primary hidden weight gain factor—false fat.

Fight Fat After Forty
Pamela Peeke, M.D., M.P.H.
ISBN 0-14-100181-X
Penguin, 2001

In Dr. Peeke's seminal work you will learn about another hidden weight gain factor—stress—and how to overcome it through lifestyle changes.

The Glucose Revolution
Jennie Brand-Miller, Ph.D., et al.
ISBN 1-56924-660-2
Marlowe & Company, 1999

This is a wonderful book that provides the most updated glycemic index and explains why foods are typed the way they are.

The New Whole Food Encyclopedia
Rebecca Wood
ISBN 0-14025-032-8
Penguin, 1999

The New Whole Foods Encyclopedia provides information on how to prepare, store, and use medicinally more than 1000 common and uncommon whole foods. Rebecca truly knows her stuff and is one of the finest natural-foods cooks I have ever had the pleasure to dine with.

Immunotics
Robert Collins Rountree, M.D., and Carol Colman
ISBN 0-399-527060
Perigree, 2001

Immunotics describes the latest nutraceuticals that dramatically increase immune function.

Antioxidant Revolution
Kenneth H. Cooper, M.D.
ISBN 0-78527-525-8
Thomas Nelson, 1997

A truly revolutionary book from the man who coined the term *aerobics*. You will be amazed to learn how overexercise can be a killer because of antioxidant depletion in the body.

Natural Hormone Balance for Women
Uzzi Reiss, M.D., with Martin Zucker
ISBN 0-74-340665-6
Pocket Books, 2000

One of the best guides to natural hormone therapy I have read. Bring this (with my own *Before the Change*, of course) to your doctor.

Dr. Atkins' Age-Defying Diet Revolution
Robert C. Atkins, M.D.
ISBN 0-131297-701-8
St. Martins Mass Market Paper, 1999

World-renowned medical expert Robert C. Atkins presents the reasons why we age and how to combat it naturally.

Caffeine Blues
Stephen Cherniske, M.S.
ISBN 0-44667-391-9
Warner Books, 1998

Cherniske is the first author to expose the dark side of America's number one drug: caffeine.

The Salt Solution
Herb Boynton, Mark F. McCarty, and Richard D. Moore, M.D., Ph.D.
ISBN 1-58333-085-2
Avery, 2001

This book contains a complete nine-step program to help you reduce salt, increase potassium, and dramatically reduce the risk of salt-induced diseases.

Healing Power of Minerals, Special Nutrients, and Trace Elements
Paul Bergner
ISBN 0-76151-021-4
Prima Publishing, 1997

Readers can find out why and how to restore essential nutrients to their diet with this informative guide.

Lights Out: Sleep, Sugar, and Survival
T.S. Wiley, Bent Formby, Ph.D. (Contributor)
ISBN 0671038680
Pocket Books, 2001

Learn how light—not just what we eat or whether we exercise—can cause obesity as well as diabetes, heart disease, and cancer.

Living Well with Hypothyroidism:
What Your Doctor Tells You . . . That You Need to Know
Mary J. Shomon
ISBN 0380808986
William Morrow and Company, 2000

Because the symptoms of hypothyroidism mimic so many other conditions (e.g., chronic fatigue, PMS, or clinical depression), learning how to deal with the underlying causes of a malfunctioning thyroid gland can put you on the right health track.

Solved: The Riddle of Illness
Stephen E. Langer, M.D., and James F. Scheer
ISBN 0658002937
McGraw-Hill, 2000

Fully updated, this classic work presents simple, effective ways to manage your thyroid and make the most of life.

Hormone Deception
D. Lindsey Berkson
ISBN 0809225387
McGraw-Hill, 2000

Find out how hormones from a variety of synthetic sources are upsetting body chemistry.

The Carnitine Miracle
Robert Crayhon, M.S.
ISBN 0871318849
M. Evans and Company, 1998

Crayhon's book explains how the supernutrient carnitine will help you to lose weight, increase energy, and lower cholesterol and triglycerides, as well as treat a wide range of health problems, including PMS, chronic fatigue, Alzheimer's and Parkinson's diseases, and many other ailments.

Know Your Fats: The Complete Primer for Understanding the Nutrition of Fats, Oils and Cholesterol
Mary G. Enig, Ph.D.
ISBN 0967812607
Bethesda Press, 2000

One of the best in-depth discussions of the many aspects of dietary fats and oils in our food and in our bodies.

Fit Happens
Joanie Greggains and Patricia Romanowski
ISBN 0375500367
Random House, 1998

This book captures Joanie's ability to get you psyched and motivated to follow her easy and fun plan for becoming thinner, happier, and healthier.

Making the Grade on Women's Health: A National and State-by-State Report Card
National Women's Law Center, Focus on Health and Leadership for Women, Center for Clinical Epidemiology and Biostatistics, University of Pennsylvania School of Medicine, and The Lewin Group, August 2000. National Women's Law Center: 1-202-588-5180.

This book is an eye-opener for professionals in public health. It is the first of its kind to assess the overall health of women at state and national levels.

Web Sites

www.ivillage.com/diet/fitness
At this Web site you will find lots of useful health information, including a Fat Flush home page and an interactive messaging board for Fat Flushers. I try to stop by whenever I can.

www.drsears.com
This is the official Web site for Dr. Barry Sears, and this is the place where you can get Dr. Sears' pharmaceutical-grade fish oil—that I mention in this book.

www.flaxcouncil.ca
A great flax site where you will learn both general and specialized flax facts. You will even find some great flax recipes that can be adapted for Fat Flush.

FITNESS RESOURCES

Trampolines

U.S. Fitness Products
3072 Wake Forest Road
Raleigh, NC 27609
1-919-875-1900
1-919-875-8010 (fax)
sales@USFitness.com

Stamina Products
Stamina Customer Service
P.O. Box 1071
Springfield, MO 65801-1071
1-800-375-7520
1-417-889-8064 (fax)
cust-srvc@staminaproducts.com

Jumpking Trampolines
Clark and Associates
11118 Ferndale Road
Dallas, TX 75238
1-214-342-0919
1-800-488-0466

Rebounder Mini Trampolines
American Institute of Reboundology, Inc
1240 East 800 North
Orem, UT 84097
1-800-464-5867
1-801-426-4509
1-801-426-9926 (fax)

COMPOUNDING PHARMACIES

While it is true that most pharmacies no longer practice compounding of prescriptions on a personal basis, I am delighted to provide a list of pharmacies that still do. Some even provide a referral listing of doctors who use natural hormone remedies for prescriptions. However, if you prefer to locate a pharmacy closer to home, you can call the International Academy of Compounding Pharmacists in Sugarland, Texas, at 800-927-4227. They will assist you in locating a local pharmacy that specializes in compounding natural prescriptions.

Wellness Health & Pharmaceuticals
2800 South 18th Street
Birmingham, AL 35209
1-800-227-2627

Triad Compounding Pharmacy
11090 East Artesia Blvd., Suite H
Cerritos, CA 90703
1-800-851-7900

Home Link National Pharmacy
381 Van Ness Blvd., Suite 1507
Torrance, CA 90501
1-888-454-8935

Oaks Pharmacy
4940 Van Nuys Blvd.
Sherman Oaks, CA 91403
1-818-990-3784

Eddie's Pharmacy
8500 Melrose Avenue
West Hollywood, CA 90069
1-310-358-2400

College Pharmacy
3505 Austin Bluffs Pkwy.
Suite 101

Colorado Springs, CO 80918
1-800-888-9358

Trumarx Drugs
501 Gordon Avenue
Thomasville, GA 31792
1-800-552-9997

Professional Arts Pharmacy
1101 North Rolling Road
Baltimore, MD 21225
1-800-832-9285

Diplomat Pharmacy
3426 Flushing Road
Flint, MI 48504
1-810-732-8720

Rocky Mountain Pharmacy
25 North Wilson Ave
Apartment C
Bozeman, MT 59715
1-406-587-4332

The Apothecary
35 Main Street
Keene, NH 03431
1-603-357-0200

Wedgewood Village Pharmacy
373 K Egg Harbor Road
Sewell, NJ 08080
1-609-589-4200

Kronus/Medical Center Compounding Pharmacy
3675 S. Rainbow
Las Vegas, NV
1-800-723-7455

Apthorp Pharmacy
2201 Broadway
New York, NY 10024
1-212-877-3480

Hospital Discount Pharmacy
104 South Bryant
Edmonds, OK 73034
1-405-348-1677

Delk Pharmacy
1602 Hatcher Lane
Columbia, TN 38401
1-616-388-3952

The Medicine Shoppe
1567 North Eastman Road
Kingsport, TN 37664
1-423-245-1022

Apothecure
13720 Midway Road
Suite 109
Dallas, TX 75244
1-800-969-6601

Greenpark Pharmacy
7515 South Main, Suite 150
Houston, TX 77030
1-713-795-5812

Belegrove Pharmacy
1535 116th Avenue Northeast
Bellevue, WA 98004
1-800-446-2123

MedQuest Pharmacy
6965 Union Park Center, Suite 100
Midville, UT 84047
1-888-222-2956

Health Pharmacy
4233 West Beltline Highway
Madison, WI 53771
1-800-373-6704

Madison Pharmacy Associates or Women's Health America
1289 Deming Way
P.O. Box 259690
Madison, WI 53717
1-800-558-7046

Women's International Pharmacy
5708 Monona Drive
Madison, WI 53716
1-800-279-5708

GRASS-FED RESOURCES

http://texasgrassfedbeef.com

You can now order grass-fed beef directly from the Internet. Choose from starter packs, value packs, and variety packs of your favorite cuts of beef!

United States

The following resources are listed by state. For the most part, these suppliers do not ship out or deliver. They are available for local sales only.

Goose Pond Farm
Charles and Laura Ritch
298 Goose Pond Road
Hartselle, AL 35640
1-256-751-0987

Pastured, free-range hens (chicken, turkey, and eggs) and grass-fed beef and lamb, free of hormones and antibiotics.

Ervin's Natural Beef
128 East 19th Street
Safford, AZ 85546
1-520-428-0033
www.ervins.com

Grass-fed beef, free of hormones, antibiotics, and pesticides.

Karen's Cimarron Ranch Natural Meats
Karen Riggs
HCR 2, Box 7152
Willcox, AZ 85643
Cimarron@vtc.net

Pastured chicken and grass-fed beef.

Blue Mountain Farm
The Elliott Family
P.O. Box 76
Fox, AR 72051
1-870-746-4704
bluemtn@aristotle.net

Pastured poultry (chicken, turkeys, and eggs)—whole, half, breast, legs, thighs, and livers.

Hosanna Hills Farm
Sam and Camie Ward
406 Ward Road
Eureka Springs, AR 72631
1-501-253-5649
sward@ipa.net

Pasture-finished beef and pastured pork.

Rivendell Gardens
Gordon and Susan Watkins
HCR 72, Box 34
Parthenon, AR 72666
1-870-446-5783
gwatkins@jasper.yournet.com

Pastured, organic chickens (June–November), turkeys (June, mid-October, November), and pigs, along with pasture-finished beef (November).

Waterfall Hollow Farm
Dave and Lisa Reeves
5854 Highway 21 South
Berryville, AR 72616
1-870-423-3457
H2ofall@cswnet.com
www.waterfallhollow.com

USDA-inspected pasture-finished beef and lamb and pastured poultry and eggs.

Bodega Pastures Sheep
Hazel Flett
Box 377
Bodega, CA 94922
jmortenson@envirolink.org
www.iplex.com/cgibin/var/iplex/adler/wool/wool.html

Grass-fed lamb.

Napa Natural Beef
10 Valley West Circle
Napa, CA 94558
1-707-255-4496
www.napanaturalbeef.com

Grass-finished Angus beef.

Rafter "S" High Ranch Country Beef
Mike and Linda Sawyer

P.O. Box 334
Bieber, CA 96009
1-530-294-5285
rafters@hdo.net

Grass-fed beef (year round) and lamb (fall).

T. O. Cattle Company
Joe and Julie Morris
500 Mission Vineyard Road
San Juan Bautista, CA 95045
tocc@compuserve.com

Split halves of grass-fed beef.

Fox Fire Farms
Richard and Linda Parry
5733 County Road 321
Ignacio, CO 81137
1-970-563-4675
foxfirefarms@frontier.net
www.foxfirefarms.com

Free-range lambs raised on grass and clover pasture, free of hormones, fertilizers, antibiotics, and pesticides.

The James Ranches
David and Kay James
33800 Highway 550
Durango, CO 81301
1-970-247-8836
jamesranch@frontier.net

Grass-fed beef, pastured poultry, and free-range eggs.

The Johnson Ranch
Clyde, Janice, and Joel Johnson
2823 Junction Street
Durango, CO 81301
1-970-247-0225

Grass-fed beef, free of antibiotics, hormones, and vaccinations.

Lasater Grasslands Beef, LLC
Matheson, CO 80830
1-719-541-2855
lasater@rmi.net
www.lasatergrasslandsbeef.com

Pasture-intensive beef cattle, free of hormones, antibiotics, and animal by-products.

Stillroven Farm
The Gurtlers
17629 Weld County Road 5
Berthoud, CO 80513
1-970-535-4527

Grass-fed beef and pastured chicken and pheasants, free of chemicals. Products available at the farm on weekends during the winter months, as well as Wednesdays and Fridays during the spring and summer months.

Lake Oriole Ranch
Dennis Stoltzfoos
8483 Croom Rital Road
Brooksville, FL 34602
1-352-799-1264

Grass-fed beef and eggs from pastured hens.

Joy-of-Illinois
1689 CR 400E
RR3
Champaign, IL 61821
1-217-863-2758

Small family farm that offers pasture-raised chickens, lambs, and ducks, free of hormones and antibiotics, in limited quantities.

The Gunthorps' Farm
Greg Gunthorp
LaGrange, IN 46761
1-219-367-2708
Hey4hogs@kuntrynet.com

Pastured pigs and chickens, free of antibiotics, stimulants, and chemicals.

J. L. Hawkins Family Farm
10373 North 300 EN
Manchester, IN 46962
1-219-982-4961
jlhawkins@kconline.com

Grass-fed beef and pastured chickens.

Organic Grass Farm
Melvin and Suvilla Fisher

RR2
Box 244-A
Rockville, IN 47872
1-765-569-5107

Grass-fed chickens, turkeys, and veal, as well as eggs from pastured poultry.

Canaan Sheep and Timber
Randall Ney
1006 Dogwood
Wellman, IA 52356
1-319-646-6696
Randall-ney@uiowa.edu

Grass-fed lamb.

Jako, Inc.
Kenneth King
6003 East Eales Road
Hutchinson, KS 67501
1-316-663-1470
kjking@mindspring.com
www.jakoinc.com

Jako is one of the few grass-only dairies in the United States (the milk has high amounts of omega-3s and CLA). Their grass-fed cattle are free of hormones, antibiotics, and additives. Pastured chickens and beef are also available.

Morrisons Grassroots Beef
David and Beth Morrison
1717 East Stimmel Road
Salina, KS 67401
1-785-823-8454
morrisonbd@informatics.net

Purely grass-fed beef and beef finished with a moderate amount of grain from cattle free of hormones and antibiotics.

Renaissance Farms
Judy and Bill Decker
1800 East 18th
Emporia, KS 66801
1-313-343-6757
anagenao@valu-line.net

Pastured Galloway beef (Scottish breed), pastured chickens, and free-range eggs.

Au Naturel Farm
Paul and Alison Wiediger
3298 Fairview Church Road
Smiths Grove, KY 42171
1-270-749-4600
awiediger@Hart.k12.ky.us

Grass-fed beef, pastured poultry (June–September), as well as free-range eggs (mid-February–October).

Harding Farms
Kelly and Anita Harding
12329 Woodsboro Road
Thurmont, MD 21788
1-301-845-7916
hrdingfrms@aol.com
http://members/aol.com/hrdingfrms

Pastured beef, eggs, chicken, turkey, and pork.

Holterholm Farms
Ron and Kathy Holter
5619A Holter Road
Jefferson, MD 21755-8508
1-301-371-4255
rwholter@aol.com

Pasture-finished beef, free of antibiotics and hormones, from Jersey and Jersey-Angus crosses.

Ruth Ann's Garden Style Beef
Ruth Ann and Steve Derrenbacher
11051 Renner Road
Woodsboro, MD 21798
1-301-898-7006
derren@cleanweb.net

Grass-fed beef.

Earth Shine Farm
Laura Kay Jones
9580 New Lothrop Road
Durand, MI 48429
1-517-288-2421

Pastured poultry products.

Oak Moon Farm
Jack Knorek
22544 20 Mile Road
Olivet, MI 49076
1-616-781-3415
knorek@internet1.net

Grass-fed beef, lamb, and pork, as well as pastured chicken, turkey, and eggs.

Dutch Mill Farm
Douglas and Janet Gunnink
25303 461 Avenue
Gaylord, MN 55334
1-507-237-5162
dgunnink@prairie.lakes.com

Grass-finished beef and lamb.

Earth-Be-Glad-Farm
Mike, Jennifer, and Johanna Rupprecht
RR2
Box 81
Lewiston, MN 55952
1-507-523-2564

Pasture-finished beef, free-range chickens, and free-range eggs, free of hormones, antibiotics, and growth promoters.

Liberty Land & Livestock
Connie Karstens and Doug Rathke
61231 MN Highway 7
Hutchinson, MN 55350
1-320-587-6094
Lambshop@hutchtel.net

Grass-fed lamb and pastured chicken, turkey, and eggs.

Shareef Family Pastured Poultry
Alvin, Abddul-Hakim, and Rosa Shareef
15 Al-Quddus Road
Sumrall, MS 39482
1-601-736-0136

Pastured poultry, sheep, and eggs, free of antibiotics, hormones, and drugs. Organic fruits and vegetables also may be available.

Crocket Beefmasters
23803 Lawrence 2140
Marionville, MO 65705
1-417-258-7251

Grass-fed beef, free of pesticides, herbicides, hormones, and antibiotics.

Green Hills Harvest
Kerry and Barb Buchmayer
14649 Highway M
Purdin, MO 64674
1-660- 244-5858

Organic milk from Jersey cows that is hormone- and pesticide-free.

The Semper Fidelis Ranch
Matthew and Albert Hempel
Route 1
Box 52
Eldridge, MO 65463
1-573-363-5213

Pasture-raised beef, pork, and chickens, free of hormones and antibiotics.

Ross Peak Ranch
Charles M. Howe
8360 Springhill Community Road
Belgrade, MT 59714
1-406-586-8884

Pasture-raised beef. Sold locally in Bozeman at Montana Harvest, Oak Street Natural Market, and The Community Food Coop and in Livingston at Food Works.

Thirteen Mile Farm
Becky Weed and David Tyler
13000 Springhill Road
Belgrade, MT 59714
1-406-388-4945
weedlamb@imt.net

Grass-fed lamb, free of hormones, antibiotics, and supplements.

The Grain Place, Inc.
Michael R. Herman
1904 North Highway
Marquette, NE 68854
1-402-854-3195

Pasture-raised beef or beef finished on grain for 30, 60, and 90 days (you get to choose).

The Perfect "10" Buffalo Ranch
Dave Hutchinson
HC 75
Box 146
Rose, NE 68772
1-402-273-4574
buffalo@bloomnet.com
www.thebuffalomarket.com

Grass-finished bison.

Tar Box Hollow Buffalo Ranch
Rose Mason
57957 871 Street Road
Dixon, NE 68732
1-402-584-2337

Bison raised on grass and grass-finished bison meat.

The Tucker Hill Farm
Bev and Chuck Henkel
1614 North 61st
Norfolk, NE 68701
1-402-371-5787
bchenkel@conpoint.com

Grass-finished beef and lamb (February–April) and pastured chickens and turkeys (June–October), free of hormones and antibiotics.

Freeman Homestead
Keith and Rae Ellen Freeman
1355 28th Creek Road
Kennedy, NY 14747
1-716-287-2056

Grass-fed beef, lamb, and pork, as well as pastured chicken and turkeys and free-range eggs.

Oswego County Beef Producers
Cornell Cooperative Extension of Oswego County
3288 Main Street
Mexico, NY 13114
1-315-963-7286

Organization of grass-fed beef producers in upstate New York. Please call or write for more information.

Sap Bush Hollow Farm
Adele and Jim Hayes
HCR 1
Box 152
Warnerville, NY 12187
1-518-234-2105
sapbush@aol.com

Pasture-raised chicken, beef, lamb, turkey, and pork, free of hormones and antibiotics.

Sweet Grass Farm
Wendy Gornick
5537 Cooper Street
Vernon, NY 13476
1-315-829-5437
wgornick@borg.com

Grass-fed lamb, pork, veal, and eggs.

ZuZu Petal's Farm
Pam Millar
439 Dawson Hill
Spencer, NY 14883
1-607-589-4762
millarjs@clarityconnect.net

Pastured poultry and hens, as well as grass-finished lamb and beef.

McNutt Farm
6120 Cutler Lake Road
Blue Rock, OH 43720
1-740-674-4555

Cattle raised on open pasture and fed grass hay in the winter months, free of hormones and antibiotics.

CMS Sheep Company
Scott and Margaret Sublette
1099 Elkhead Road
Yoncalla, OR 97499
1-541-849-2871
sublette@wanweb.net

Fall lambs are fed small amounts of grain in addition to grass, and spring lambs are finished on clover and grass only. Pastured pork available in the fall. Limited supply of beef available from Jersey cows or dairy cross calves butchered in June after grazing on spring grass.

The Graf Century Farm
Nita and Loren Wilton
44222 Southeast Louden Road
Corbett, OR 97019
1-503-695-5452

Pasture-finished beef and pastured chickens and turkeys.

Kneedeep Grass & Cattle Company
Ken and Connie Pond
302 Southwest 23rd Street
Hermiston, OR 97838
1-541-567-4470
pondk@oregontrail.net

Grass-finished beef and pastured chicken and turkeys.

River Run Farm
James and Ellen Girt
19224 Swedetown Road
Clatskanie, OR 97016
1-503-728-4561
egirt@aone.com

Organic, pasture-finished beef from Black Angus cattle. Sold at the Portland Farmer's Market.

Canyon Livestock Company
RD 6
Box 205
Wellsboro, PA 16901
1-570-724-7788

Pasture-finished and grass-fed beef.

Double G Farm
Barb and Ken Gorski
227 Henne Road
Bernville, PA 19506
1-610-488-6555

Pastured poultry and eggs from pastured hens.

Dr. Elkins' Angusburger
3575 Doe Run Church Road
East Fallowfield, PA 19320
1-610-486-0789
elkins32@aol.com

Most meat is pure ground beef made from Angus steers, pasture-raised and free of hormones and antibiotics.

Forks Farm
The Hopkins Family
299 Covered Bridge Rd.
Orangeville, PA 17859
1-570-683-5820
forks@epics.net

Pasture-finished beef, pastured pork, grass-finished lamb, and pastured chicken and turkey.

Marwood Farm
Donald and Christine Scott
1068 Woodstock
Fayetteville, PA 17222
1-717-352-7090

Free-range eggs, pastured chicken and turkey, and grass-fed beef. Also have pasture-finished beef.

Overlook Farm
Rob and Alanna Reed
233 Spruce Road
Karns City, PA 16041
1-724-756-0540

Grass-fed beef, free of hormones and antibiotics.

Things Eternal Farm
Randy Simpson
3489 Bullfrog Road
Fairfield, PA 17320
1-717-642-6450
bullfrog@wideopen.net

Pastured poultry and pork.

WIL-AR Farms
Wilmer and Arlene Newswanger
76 Parker Road
Newville, PA 17241
1-717-776-6552

Small family farm with limited amounts of grass-fed beef, veal, lamb, pork, chicken, turkey, eggs, butter, yogurt, and cream.

Crusader Farms
P.O. Box 1312
Anderson, SC 29622
1-864-296-4541

Pastured chickens, turkeys, lamb, and beef and free-range eggs.

Greenbrier Farms
John and Joyce Palmer
772 Hester Store Road
Easley, SC 29640
1-888-859-0125

Free-range Senepol-Angus cross beef cattle, free of hormones and antibiotics.

Peaceful Pastures All Natural Meats
Darrin and Jenny Drake
69 Cowan Valley Lane
Hickman, TN 38567
1-615-683-5556
peacepast@aol.com

Chicken, turkey, pork, lamb (pasture-raised), dairy goats (some grain), veal (some grain), and beef (some grain).

Homestead Healthy Foods
Richard and Peggy Sechrist
Route 2
Box 184-A
Fredericksburg, TX 78624
1-888-861-5670
www.homesteadhf.com

Pastured, certified organic, grass-fed beef and chicken. Chickens are fed a feed ration that contains organic flaxseed oil, a source of omega-3 fatty acids.

Slanker's Grass Fed Meats
Chris Slanker
RR2
Box 175
Powderly, TX 75473
1-866-752-6537
1-903-732-4653
goodmeat@slanker.com
http://texasgrassfedbeef.com

Just 100 percent pasture-finished beef.

The Texas Bison Company
Jan and Austin Moseley
3582 County Road 2150
Caddo Mills, TX 75135
1-903-527-2325
jmoseley@webwide.net
www.bisonranch.com

Grass-finished bison, free of hormones and antibiotics.

Ensign Ranches
Gregg Simonds
6315 North Snowview Drive
Park City, UT 84086
1-435-647-9134
jsimonds@uswest.net

Large cattle and wildlife operation with grass-fed beef.

Meadow Creek Dairy
The Feete Family
6380 Meadow Creek Road
Galax, VA 24333
mcd@ls.net
www.ls.net/!mcd

Practice management-intensive grazing with herd of Jersey cows, free of herbicides and pesticides.

Pearce and Lori Gardner
558 Bowlers Road
Tappahannock, VA 22560
1-804-443-1010
gpromo@access.digex.net

Pastured veal and pork, as well as broilers and eggs.

Polyface, Inc.
The Salatins
Route 1
Box 281
Swoope, VA 24479
1-540-885-3590

Free-range hens and pastured beef, chicken, turkey, and pigs, free of fertilizers, pesticides, and herbicides.

Thorntree Farm
Route 2
Box 776A
Nickelsville, VA 24271
1-540-479-3422

Cattle raised on grass without hormones or antibiotics.

Weatherbury Station
RR3, Box 767
Tazewell, VA 24651
1-276-472-2535
(fax) 1-276-472-2536
gswhitted@inetone.net

Grass-fed lamb, as well as pastured poultry and eggs from free-range hens.

The Flack Family Farm
RD 2
Box 900
Enosburg Falls, VT 05450
1-802-933-7752
bflack@lamoille.k12.vt.us
www.together.net/~bflack

Pasture-raised and -finished lamb.

The Hill Farm of Vermont
Peter Young and Nancy Everhart
RD 1
Box 740
Plainfield, VT 05667
1-802-426-3234

Organically certified, pasture-raised beef.

Oyster Bay Farm
4931 Oyster Bay Road Northwest
Olympia, WA 98502
1-360-866-9424

Lamb from animals fed small amounts of grain.

Cattleana Ranch
Thomas and Susan Wychota
5200 O'Reilly Road
Omro, WI 54963
1-920-685-6964

Pasture-finished Galloway beef and free-range chickens.

Northstar Bison
1936 28th Avenue
Rice Lake, WI 54868
1-715-234-9085
www.northstarbison.com

Grass-fed bison.

Four Winds Farm
Juliet Tomkins
N8806 600th Street
River Falls, WI 54022
1-715-425-6037
4winds@win.bright.net

Pasture-raised beef, pork, and chicken.

Snowy Fields Farm
407 310 Street
Wilson, WI 54027
1-715-772-3175
ficken@win.bright.net

Beef, lamb, pork, veal, and chickens, free of hormones or antibiotics.

Canada

Deer Creek Ranch
Neal Gilchrist and Dr. Susan Lea
Box 86
Milk River, AB T0K 1M0 Canada
1-403-647-3644
swtgrass@telusplanet.net

Grass-finished beef.

Sunwords Farm
Box 55
Armena, AB T0B 0G0 Canada
1-877-393-3133
sunwords@telusplanet.net

Pastured poultry, free of additives and hormones.

Dave and Pat Griffith
Box 1942
Vanderhoof, BC V0J 3A0 Canada
1-250-567-2860
ebus292@uniserve.com

Pasture-raised chickens, turkeys, pigs, and cattle, free of hormones, pesticides, and herbicides.

Mother Nature's Beef
M. Masserini
P.O. Box 34
Lake Francis, MB R0C 1T0 Canada
(fax) 1-204-383-5828
ml.masserini@wanadoo.fr

Grass-fed beef and beef finished on grain.

Webers' Pasture Farm
Marvin and Amanda Weber
RR2
Dobbinton, ON N0H 1L0 Canada
1-519-934-9906

Pasture-finished beef, grass-fed lamb, pastured pork, pastured chickens, and eggs from free-range hens.

Daleview Farm
John and Karen Dale
Box 75
Meacham, SK S0K 2V0 Canada
1-306-944-4241

Grass-fed beef, pork, and poultry.

References

PREFACE

Finn, S. C. "Helping Women Find Everyday Solutions." *J Womens Health Gender-Based Med* 9:9(2000):951–954.
Gittleman, A. L. *Beyond Pritikin*. New York: Bantam, 1988.
Louden, J. *The Woman's Comfort Book*. New York: HarperSan Francisco, 1992, pp. 1–2.
"Women's Health Issues Survey." *Wirthlin Worldwide* (October 1999).

CHAPTER 1

Anderson, K. E., and Kappas, A. "Dietary Regulation of Cytochrome P-450." *Annu Rev Nutr* 11(1991):141–167.
Bland, J. S. *The 20-Day Rejuvenation Diet Program*. Los Angeles: Keats, 1999.
Bland, J. S. "Food and Nutrient Effects on Detoxification." *Townsend Letter for Doctors* (December 1995).
Bland, J. S., and Bralley, J. A. "Nutritional Up-Regulation of Hepatic Detoxification Enzymes." *J Appl Nutr* 3–4(1992):2–15.
Bock, K. *The Road to Immunity: How to Survive and Thrive in a Toxic World*. New York: Pocket Books, 1997.
Breecher, M. "A Natural Aid to Weight Reduction for the Chronically Fat." *Let's Live Magazine* (August 1982):70–73.
Brush, M. G., Watson, S. J., Horrobin, D. F., and Manku, M. S. "Abnormal Essential Fatty Acid Levels in Plasma of Women with Premenstrual Syndrome." *Am J Obstet Gynecol* 150(1984):363–366.
Cabot, S. *The Liver Cleansing Diet*. Scottsdale, AZ: SCB International, 1999.
Caldwell, J., and Jakoby, W. B. *Biological Basis of Detoxification*. New York: Academic Press, 1983.
Charalambous, B. M. "Erythrocyte Sodium Pump Activity in Human Obesity." *Clin Chim Acta* 141:2–3(1984):179–187.
Galland, L. *The Four Pillars of Healing*. New York: Random House, 1997.
Gittleman, A. L. *Beyond Pritikin*. New York: Bantam, 1988.
Gittleman, A. L. *Super Nutrition for Women*. New York: Bantam, 1991.
Haslett, C., et al. "A Double Blind Evaluation of Evening Primrose Oil as an Anti-Obesity Agent." *Int J Obesity* 7(1983):549–553.

Haas, E. *The Detox Diet*. Millbrae, CA: Celestial Arts, 1996.
Heaton, J. M. "The Distribution of Brown Adipose Tissue in the Human." *J Anat* 112(1972):35.
Heleniak, E. P., and Aston, B. "Prostaglandins, Brown Fat, and Weight Loss." *Med Hypoth* 28(1989):13–33.
Henry, C. J., and Emery, B. "Effect of Spiced Food on Metabolic Rate." *Hum Nutr Clin Nutr* 40:2(1986):165–168.
Himms-Hagen, J. "Obesity May Be Due to a Malfunctioning of Brown Fat." *Can Med Assoc J* 121(1976):1361–1364.
Horrobin, D.F. "The Role of Essential Fatty Acids and Prostaglandins in the Premenstrual Syndrome." *J Reprod Med* 28(1983):465–468.
Jakoby, W. B. (ed.). *Enzymatic Basis of Detoxification*, Vol II. New York: Academic Press, 1980.
Jakoby, W. B., Bend, J. R., and Caldwell, J. (eds.). *Metabolic Basis of Detoxification: Metabolism of Functional Groups*. New York: Academic Press, 1981.
Lemole, G. M. *The Healing Diet*. New York: William Morrow, 2000.
Mercer, S. W. "Effect of High Fat Diets on Energy Balance and Thermogenesis in Brown Adipose Tissue of Lean and Genetically Obese Mice." *J Nutr* 117:12 (1987):2147–2153.
Mir, M.A., et al. "Erythrocyte Sodium Potassium-ATPase Transport in Obesity." *N Engl J Med* 305(1981):1264–1268.
Sears, B. *The Zone*. New York: Regan Books, 1995.
Takada, R., Saitoh, M., and Mori, T. "Dietary γ-Linolenic Acid-Enriched Oil Reduces Body Fat Content and Induces Liver Enzyme Activities Relating to Fatty Acid β Oxidation in Rats." *J Nutr* 124(1994):469–474.
Vadaddi, K. S., and Horrobin, D. F. "Weight Loss Produced by Evening Primrose Oil Administered in Normal and Schizophrenic Individuals." *IRCS J Med Sci* 7(1979):52–55.
"Why You Need to Protect Your Liver." *Consumer Reports on Health* 13:4(April 2001):6–9.

CHAPTER 2

Hidden Factor #1: Your Tired, Toxic Liver

Anderson, J. W., et al. "Long-Term Cholesterol-Lowering Effects of Psyllium as an Adjunct to Diet Therapy in the Treatment of Hypercholesterolemia." *Am J Clin Nutr* 71:6(2000):1433–1438.
Anderson, J. W., et al. "Effects of Psyllium on Glucose and Serum Lipid Responses in Men with Type II Diabetes and Hypercholesterolemia." *Am J Clin Nutr* 70:4(1999):466–473.
Arrigoni-Martelli, E., and Caso, V. "Carnitine Protects Mitochondria and Removes Toxic Acyls from Xenobiotics." *Drugs Exp Clin Res* 27:1(2001):27–49.

Asai, A., Nakagawa, K., and Miyazawa, T. "Antioxidative Effects of Turmeric, Rosemary, and Capsicum Extracts on Membrane Phospholipid Peroxidation and Liver Lipid Metabolism in Mice." *Biosci Biotechnol Biochem* 63:12(1999):2118–2122.

Berdanier, C. D. "Inositol: An Essential Nutrient?" *Nutrition Today* 27(1992):22–26.

Brevetti, G., et al. "Changes in Skeletal Muscle Histology and Metabolism in Patients Undergoing Exercise Reconditioning: Effect of Proprionyl-L-Carnitine." *Muscle Nerve* 20(1997):1115–1120.

Cabot, S. *The Liver Cleansing Diet*. Scottsdale, AZ: SCB International, 1996.

Chen, H., Zuo, Y., and Deng, Y. "Separation and Determination of Flavonoids and Other Phenolic Compounds in Cranberry Juice by High-Performance Liquid Chromatography." *J Chromatogr A* 913:1–2(2001):387–395.

Cherniske, S. *Caffeine Blues*. New York: Warner Books, 1998.

Crayhon, R. *The Carnitine Miracle*. New York: Evans and Company, 1998.

Cunnane, S. C., et al. "Nutritional Attributes of Traditional Flaxseed in Healthy Young Adults." *Am J Clin Nutr* 61:1(1995):62–68.

Dayanandan, A., Kumar, P., and Panneerselvam, C. "Protective Role of L-Carnitine on Liver and Heart Lipid Peroxidation in Atherosclerotic Rats." *J Nutr Biochem* 12:5(2001):254–257.

Delergy, H. J., et al. "Effects of Amount and Type of Dietary Fiber on Short-Term Control of Appetite." *Int J Food Sci Nutr* 48:1(1997):67–77.

Dyck, D. J. "Dietary Fat Intake, Supplements, and Weight Loss." *Can J Appl Physiol* 25:6(2000):495–523.

Eldershaw, T. P., et al. "Pungent Principles of Ginger (*Zingiber officinale*) Are Thermogenic in the Perfused Rat Hindlimb." *Int J Obesity Related Metabol Disord* 16:10(1992):755–763.

Facchinetti, F., et al. "Oral Magnesium Successfully Relieves Premenstrual Mood Changes." *Obstet Gynecol* 78:2(1991):177–181.

Flora, K., et al. "Milk Thistle (*Silybum marianum*) for the Therapy of Liver Disease." *Am J Gastroenterol* 94:2(1999):545–546.

Gittleman, A. L. *The Living Beauty Detox Program*. New York: HarperSan Francisco, 2000.

Hahn, P., and Skala, J. "The Role of Carnitine in Brown Adipose Tissue of Suckling Rats." *Comp Biochem Physiol* 51B(1975):507.

Hamadeh, M. J., et al. "Nutritional Aspects of Flaxseed in the Human Diet." *Proc Flax Inst* 4(1992):48–53.

Hu, F. B., et al. "A Prospective Study of Egg Consumption and Risk of Cardiovascular Disease in Men and Women." *JAMA* 281:15(1999):1387–1394.

Imparl-Radosevich, J., et al. "Regulation of PTP-1 and Insulin Receptor Kinase by Fractions from Cinnamon: Implications for Cinnamon Regulation of Insulin Signaling." *Horm Res* 50:3(1998):177–182.

Jenkins, D. J., et al. "Effect of Psyllium in Hypercholesterolemia at Two Monounsaturated Fatty Acid Intakes." *Am J Clin Nutr* 65:5(1997):1524–1533.

Lake, R. *Liver Cleansing Handbook.* Vancouver, Canada: Alive Books, 2000.

Langner, E., et al. "Ginger: History and Use." *Adv Ther* 15:1(1998):25–44.

Lebowitz, B. "Carnitine." *J Opt Nutr* 22(1993):90–109.

Mickelfied, G. H., et al. "Effects of Ginger on Gastroduodenal Motility." *Int J Clin Pharmacol Ther* 37:7(1999):341–346.

Mills, S. Y. *Out of the Earth: The Essential Book of Herbal Medicine.* London: Penguin Books, 1991, p. 282.

Murray, M. T., and Pizzorno, J. *Encyclopedia of Natural Medicine.* Rocklin, CA: Prima Publishing, 1991, pp. 51–56.

Olson, B. H., et al. "Psyllium-Enriched Cereals Lower Blood Total Cholesterol and LDL Cholesterol, but Not HDL Cholesterol, in Hypercholesterolemic Adults: Results of a Meta-Analysis." *J Nutr* 127:10(1997):1973–1980.

Park, B. K., and Kirreringham, N.R. "Assessment of Enzyme Induction and Enzyme Inhibition in Humans: Toxicological Implications." *Xenobiotica* 20:11(1990):1339–1343.

Pepping, J. "Milk Thistle: *Silybum marianum.*" *Am J Health Syst Pharm* 56:12(1999):1196–1197.

Raczkotilla, E., et al. "The Action of *Taraxacum officinale* Extracts on the Body Weight Diuresis of Laboratory Animals." *Planta Med* 26(1974):212–217.

Rutherford, P. P, and Deacon, A. C. "The Mode of Action of Dandelion Root Fructofuranosideases on Insulin." *Biochem J* 129:2(1972):511–512.

Salmi, H. A., et al. "Effect of Silymarin on Chemical, Functional, and Morphological Alterations of the Liver." *Scand J Gastroenterol* 17(1982):512–517.

Shakil, A. O., et al. "Acute Liver Failure: Clinical Features, Outcome, Analysis, Applicability." *Liver Transplant* 6(2000):163–169.

Shear, N. H., et al. "Acetaminophen-Induced Toxicity to Human Epidermoid Cell Line A431 and Hepatoblastoma Cell Line: Hep G2, in Vitro, Is Diminished by Silymarin." *Skin Pharmacol* 8:6(1995):279–291.

Velussi, M., et al. "Long-Term (12 Months) Treatment with an Antioxidant Drug (Silymarin) Is Effective on Hyperinsulinemia, Exogenous Insulin Need and Malondialdehyde Levels in Cirrhotic Diabetic Patients." *J Hepatol* 26:4(1997):871–879.

"Why You Need to Protect Your Liver." *Consumer Reports on Health.* (April 2001):6–9.

Zhi-Qian, H. E., et al. "Body Weight Reduction in Adolescents by a Combination of Measures Including Using L-Carnitine." *Acta Nutr Sinica* 19:2(1997):146–151.

Hidden Factor #2: When Fat Is Not Fat

Adlercreutz, H., et al. "Inhibition of Human Aromatase by Mammalian Lignans and Isoflavonoid Phytoestrogens." *J Steroid Biochem Mol Biol* 44(1993):147–153.

Bateson-Koch, C. *Allergies: Diseases in Disguise*. Vancouver, Canada: Alive Books, 1994.

Bodel, P. T., Colran, R., and Kass, E. H. "Cranberry Juice and Antibacterial Action of Hippuric Acid." *J Lab Clin Med* 54(1959):881–888.

Braley, J. *Dr. Braley's Food Allergy and Nutrition Revolution*. New Canaan, CT: Keats Publishing, 1992.

Browder, S. E. *The Power*. New York: Wiley, 2001.

Chrohn, J. *Natural Detox: The Complete Guide to Allergy Relief and Prevention*. Point Roberts, WA: Hartley and Marks, 1996.

Crook, W. G. *Yeast Connection: A Medical Breakthrough*. Jackson, TN: Vintage Books, 1980.

Dancey, E. *The Cellulite Solution*. New York: St. Martin's Press, 1997.

De Stefani, F., et al. "Dietary Fiber and Risk of Breast Cancer: A Case-Controlled Study in Uruguay." *Nutr Cancer* 28(1997):14–19.

Espeland, M. A., et al. "Effect of Postmenopausal Hormone Therapy on Body Weight and Waist and Hip Girths: Postmenopausal Estrogen-Progestin Interventions Study Investigators." *J Clin Endocrinol Metab* 82:5(1997):1549–1556.

Gittleman, A. L. *Beyond Pritikin*. New York: Bantam Books, 1996.

Gittleman, A. L. *Eat Fat, Lose Weight*. Los Angeles: Keats, 1999.

Gottesman, R. "How Symptoms Tell the Story of Hormone Imbalance." *John Lee Med Lett* (April 1998):5–6.

Greenwood-Robinson, M. *The Cellulite Breakthrough*. New York: Dell, 2000.

Guigliano, D., Torella, R., and Sgambat, S. "Effects of Alpha- and Beta-Adrenergic Inhibition and Somatostatin on Plasma Glucose, Free Fatty Acids, Insulin, Glucagon, and Growth Hormone Responses to Prostaglandin E_1 in Man." *J Clin Endocrinol Metab* 48(1979):302.

Haas, E. M., and Stauth, C. *The False Fat Diet*. New York, Ballantine Books, 2000.

Horrobin, D. F. "The Role of Essential Fatty Acids and Prostaglandins in the Premenstrual Syndrome." *J Reprod Med* 28(1983):465–468.

Knotts, C. T., et al. "Endomesyum Antibodies in Blood Donors Predicts a High Prevalence of Celiac Disease in the United States." *J Gastroenterol* (April 1996).

Lee, Y. L., et al. "Does Cranberry Juice Have Antibacterial Activity?" *JAMA* 283:13(2000):1691.

Ofek, I., Goldhar, J., and Sharon, N. "Anti–*Escherichia coli* Adhesion Activity of Cranberry and Blueberry Juices." *Adv Exp Med Biol* 408(1996):179–183.

Papas, P.N., Brusch, C.A., and Ceresia, G. C. "Cranberry Juice in the Treatment of Urinary Tract Infections." *Southwest Med* 47(1966):17–20.

Randolph, T. G. *An Alternative Approach to Allergies*. New York: HarperCollins, 1990.

Rigaud, D., et al. "Effect of Psyllium on Gastric Emptying, Hunger Feeling and Food Intake in Normal Volunteers: A Double-Blind Study." *Eur J Clin Nutr* 52:4(1998):239–245.

Smith, I. K. "The Tylenol Scare." *Time* (April 9, 2001):81.

Thompson, L. U. "Flaxseed and its Lignan and Oil Components Reduce Mammary Tumor Growth at Late Stage of Carcinogenesis." *Carcinogenesis* 17:6(1996):1373–1376.

Walker, E. B., et al. "Cranberry Concentrate: UTI Prophylaxis." *J Fam Pract* 45:2(1997):167–168.

Wang, C., et al. "Lignans and Flavonoids Inhibit Aromatase Enzyme in Human Preadipocytes." *J Steroid Biochem Mol Biol* 50(1994):205–212.

Whitaker, J. "Should You Use HRT?" *Health Healing* 6(2001):4–8.

Yeager, S. "Banish Cellulite in Minutes." *Prevention* (June 2001):150–157.

Zava, D. "Teenage Girls, Hormone Balance and Birth Control Pills." *John Lee Med Lett* (January 1999):5–6.

Hidden Factor #3: Fear of Fat

American Chemical Society National Meeting News. "CLA Could Help Control Weight, Fat, Diabetes, and Muscle Loss," August 20, 2000.

Belury, M. A. "Role of Conjugated Linoleic Acid (CLA) in the Management of Type 2 Diabetes: Evidence from Zucker Diabetic Rats and Human Subjects." Presented at the American Chemical Society National Meeting, August 21, 2000.

Belury, M. A., and Vanden Heuval, J. P. "Protection Against Cancer and Heart Disease by the Dietary Fatty Acid, Conjugated Linoleic Acid: Potential Mechanisms of Action." *Nutr Dis Update J* 1:2(1997):53–58.

Blankson, H., et al. "Conjugated Linoleic Acid Reduces Body Fat Mass in Overweight and Obese Humans." *J Nutr* 130:12(2000):2943–2948.

Clement, I. P., and Scimeca, J. A. "Conjugated Linoleic Acid and Linoleic Acid Are Distinctive Modulators of Mammary Carcinogenesis." *Nutr Cancer* 27:2(1997):131–135.

Clement, I. P., et al. "Mammary Cancer Prevention by Conjugated Dienoic Derivative of Linoleic Acid." *Cancer Res* 51(1991):6118–6124.

Cunnane, S. C., et al. "Ω-3 Essential Fatty Acids Decrease Weight Gain in Genetically Obese Mice." *Br J Nutr* 56(1986):87–95.

Erling, T. "A Pilot Study with the Aim of Studying the Efficacy and Tolerability of Tonalin CLA on the Body Composition in Humans." Lillestrom, Norway: Medstat Research, Ltd., 1997.

Horrocks, L., and Yeo, Y. "Health Benefits of Docosahexaenoic Acid (DHA)." *Pharm Res* 40:3(1999):211–225.

Hudson, T. "The Good Fat for Women." *Health Products Bus* 29(October 2000):25–26.

Kirtland, S. J. "Prostaglandin E_1: A Review." *Prostaglandins Leukotrienes Essential Fatty Acids* 32(1988):165–174.

Lands, W. E. "Biochemistry and Physiology of Ω-3 Fatty Acids." *FASEB J* 6(1992):2530–2536.

Okuyama, H. "Dietary Fatty Acids: The ω-6/ω-3 Balance and Chronic Elderly Diseases: Excess Linoleic Acid (ω-6) and Relative ω-3 Deficiency Syndrome Seen in Japan." *Progr Lipid Res* 35:4(1997):409–457.

Pariza, M. W. "Conjugated Linoleic Acid: A Newly Recognized Nutrient." *Chemistry and Industry* (June 16, 1997):464–466.

Pariza, M. W. "The Biological Activities of Conjugated Linoleic Acid." *Adv Conj Linoleic Acid Res* 1(1999):12–20.

Pariza, M. W., Park, Y., and Cook, M. E. "Conjugated Linoleic Acid and the Control of Cancer and Obesity." *Toxicol Sci* 52(Suppl, 1999):107–110.

Park, Y., and Cook, M. E. "Mechanisms of Action of Conjugated Linoleic Acid: Evidence and Speculation." *Proc Soc Exp Biol Med* 233(2000):8–13.

Robinson , J. *Why Grassfed Is Best!* Vashon, WA: Island Press, 2000.

Siguel, E. N., Lerman, R. H. "Prevalence of Essential Fatty Acid Deficiency in Patients with Chronic Gastrointestinal Disorders." *Metabolism* 45(1996):12–23.

Simopoulos, A. "Omega-3 Fatty Acids in Health and Disease and in Growth and Development." *Am J Clin Nutr* 54(1991):438–463.

Simopoulos, A. P. "Essential Fatty Acids in Health and Chronic Disease." *Am J Clin Nutr* 70(Suppl, 1999):560S–569S.

Simopoulos, A. P., and Robinson, J. *The Omega Diet*. New York: HarperCollins, 1998.

Storlien, L. H. "Not All Dietary Fats May Lead to Obesity." *Am J Clin Nutr* 51(1990):1114.

Watkins, B. A., and Seifert, M. F. "Conjugated Linoleic Acid and Bone Biology." *J Am Coll Nutr* 19:4(2000):478–486.

Yeonhwa, P., et al. "Effect of Conjugated Linoleic Acid on Body Composition in Mice." *Lipids* 32:8(1997):853–858.

Hidden Factor #4: Excess Insulin

Anderson, R. A., et al. "Elevated Intakes of Supplemental Chromium Improve Glucose and Insulin Variables in Individuals with Type II Diabetes." *Diabetes* 46(1997):1786–1791.

Atkins, R. C., and Buff, S. *Dr. Atkin's Age-Defying Diet Revolution*. New York: St. Martin's Press, 2000.

Borkman, M., et al. "The Relation Between Insulin Sensitivity and the Fatty-Acid Composition of Skeletal-Muscle Phospholipids." *N Engl J Med* 328:4(1993):238–244.

Brand-Miller, J., et al. *The Glucose Revolution*. New York: Marlowe and Company, 1999.

Cefalu, W. T., et al. "The Effect of Chromium Supplementation on Carbohydrate Metabolism and Body Fat Distribution." *Diabetes* 46(Suppl, 1997):55A.

Challem, J., et al. *Syndrome X: The Complete Nutritional Program to Prevent and Reverse Insulin Resistance*. New York: Wiley, 2001.

Clarke, S. D., et al. "Fatty Acid Regulation of Gene Expression: Its Role in Fuel Partitioning and Insulin Resistance." *Ann N Y Acad Sci* 827(1997):178–187.

Clarksen, P. M. "Nutritional Ergogenic Aids: Chromium, Exercise, and Muscle Mass." *Int J Sport Nutr* 1(1991):289–293.

Collier, G. R., et al. "The Acute Effect of Fat on Insulin Secretion." *J Clin Endocrinol Metab* 66(1988):323–326.

Evans, G. W. "Chromium: Insulin Cohort." *Total Health* (August 1994):42–43.

Evans, G. W. *Chromium Picolinate.* Garden City, NY: Avery, 1996.

Fanaian, M., et al. "The Effect of Modified Fat Diet on Insulin Resistance and Metabolic Parameters in Type II Diabetes." *Diabetologia* 89(1996):A7.

Gittleman, A. L. *The 40/30/30 Phenomenon*. New Canaan, CT: Keats Publishing, 1997.

Gittleman, A. L. *Your Body Knows Best*. New York: Pocket Books, 1997.

Grant, P. "Does Bread Make You Fat?" *McCall's* (October 2000):100–103.

Holt, S. H., Brand-Miller, J. C., and Petocz, P. "Interrelationships among Postprandial Satiety, Glucose and Insulin Responses and Changes in Subsequent Food Intake." *Eur J Clin Nutr* 50(December 1996):788–797.

Holt, S.H., Brand-Miller, J. C., Petocz, P., and Farmakalidis, E. "A Satiety Index of Common Foods." *Eur J Clin Nutr* 49(September 1995):675–690.

Kozlovsky, A. S., et al. "Effects of Diets High in Simple Sugars on Urinary Chromium Losses." *Metabolism* 35(1986):515–518.

Lee, B. M., and Wolever, T. M. S. "Effect of Glucose, Sucrose, and Fructose on Plasma Glucose and Insulin Responses in Normal Humans: Comparison with White Bread." *Eur J Clin Nutr* 52(1998):924–928.

Levi, B., and Werman, M. G. "Long-Term Fructose Consumption Accelerates Glycation and Several Age-Related Variables in Male Rats." *J Nutr* 128:1(1998):1442–1449.

McCarty, M. F. "The Case for Supplemental Chromium and a Survey of Clinical Studies with Chromium Picolinate." *J Appl Nutr* 43(1991):58–66.

Opara, J. U., and Levine, J. H. "The Deadly Quartet: The Insulin Resistance Syndrome." *South Med J* 90(1997):1162–1168.

Provonsha, S. "A Hypothesis Regarding Meat and the Insulin-Resistant State Known as Syndrome X." *Veget Nutr* 2:3(1988):119–126.

Reaven, G. M. "Insulin Resistance, the Key to Survival: A Rose by Any Other Name." *Diabetologia* 42(1988):384–385.

Reaven, G. M. "Role of Insulin Resistance in Human Disease." *Diabetes* 37(1988):1595–1607.

Reaven, G. M. "Pathophysiology of Insulin Resistance in Human Disease." *Physiol Rev* 75(1995):473–485.

Reaven, G. M. "Hypothesis: Muscle Insulin Resistance Is the (Not So) Thrifty Genotype." *Diabetologia* 41(1998):482–484.

Rothwell, N .J., and Stock, M. J. "Insulin and Thermogenesis." *Int J Obesity* 12(1988):93–102.

Schwarz, J. M., et al. "Thermogenesis in Obese Women: Effect of Fructose vs. Glucose Added to a Meal." *Am J Physiol* 262:4 (pt 1, 1992):E394–E401.

Spieth, L. E., et al. "A Low-Glycemic Index Diet in the Treatment of Pediatric Obesity." *Arch Pediatr Adolesc Med* 154:9(2000):947–951.

Storlien, L. H., et al. "The Type of Dietary Fat Has a Profound Influence on Development of Insulin Resistance in Rats." *Diabetes Res Clin Pract* 5(Suppl 1, 1988):S267.

Torjesen, P. A., et al. "Lifestyle Changes May Reverse Development of the Insulin Resistance Syndrome." *Diabetes Care* 30(1997):26–31.

Trent, L. K., et al. "Effects of Chromium Picolinate on Body Composition." *J Sports Med Phys Fitness* 35(1995):273–280.

Van Gaal, L., et al. "Carbohydrate-Induced Thermogenesis in Obese Women: Effect of Insulin and Catecholamines." *J Endocrinol Invest* 22:2(1999):109–114.

Williams, K. V., and Korytkowski, M. T. "Syndrome X: Pathogenesis, Clinical and Therapeutic Aspects." *Diabetes Nutr Metabol* 11(1998):140–152.

Hidden Factor #5: Stress as Fat Maker

Bjorntorp, P. "Visceral Obesity: A Civil Syndrome." *Obesity Res* 1(1993):206–222.

Blackman, M. R. "Age-Related Alterations in Sleep Quality and Neuroendocrine Function: Interrelationships and Implications." *JAMA* 284:7(2000):861–868.

Browder, S. E. "Stress Busters That Can Save Your Life." *New Choices* (November 2000):41–44.

Epel, E. S., et al. "Stress-Induced Cortisol, Mood, and Fat Distribution in Men." *Obesity Res* 7:1(1999):9–15.

Epel, E. S., et al. "Stress and Body Shape: Stress-Induced Cortisol Secretion Is Consistently Greater Among Women with Central Fat." *Psychosom Med* 62:5(2000):623–632.

Epel, E. S., et al. "Stress May Add Bite to Appetite in Women: A Laboratory Study of Stress-Induced Cortisol and Eating Behavior." *Psychoneuroendocrinology* 26:1(2001):37–49.

Gaynor, M. L., and Hickey, J. *Dr. Gaynor's Cancer Prevention Program.* New York: Kensington Books, 1999.
Gray-Foltz, D. "The Relaxing Way to Lose Weight," *Health* :90–95.
"Less Fun, Less Sleep, More Work: An American Portrait," National Sleep Foundation Poll, March 27, 2001.
Peeke, P. *Fight Fat after Forty.* New York: Penguin, 2000.
Peeke, P., and Chrousos, G. P. "Hypercortisolism and Obesity." *Ann N Y Acad Sci* 77(1995):665–676.
Van Cauter, E., Leproult, R., and Plat, L. "Age-Related Changes in Slow Wave Sleep and REM Sleep and Relationship with Growth Hormone and Cortisol Levels in Healthy Men." *JAMA* 284:7(2000):879–881.
Wiley, T. S, and Formby, B. *Lights Out: Sleep, Sugar and Survival.* New York: Pocket Books, 2001.
Yudkin, J. *Sweet and Dangerous.* New York: Wyden Books, 1972.

CHAPTER 7

Exercise

Alessio, H. M., et al. "Lipid Peroxidation and Scavenger Enzymes during Exercise: Adaptive Response to Training." *J Appl Physiol* 64:4 (1988):1333–1336.
Coates, G., O'Brodovich, H., and Goeree, G. "Hindlimb and Lung Lymph Flows during Prolonged Exercise." *J Appl Physiol* 75:2(1993):633–638.
Cooper, K. H. *The Antioxidant Revolution.* Nashville, TN: Thomas Nelson, 1994.
DeSouza, C. A. "Regular Aerobic Exercise Prevents and Restores Age-Related Declines in Endothelium-Dependent Vasodilation in Healthy Men." *Circulation* 102:12(2000):1351–1357.
Fogelholm, M., et al. "Effects of Walking Training on Weight Maintenance after a Very Low-Energy Diet in Premenopausal Obese Women: A Randomized, Controlled Trial." *Arch Intern Med* 160:14(2000):2177–2184.
Gittleman, A. L. *Super Nutrition for Menopause.* Garden City, NY: Avery, 1998.
King, N. A., Tremblay, A., and Blundell, J. E. "Effects of Exercise on Appetite Control: Implications for Energy Balance." *Med Sci Sports Exerc* 29:8(1997):1076–1089.
Layne, J. E., and Nelson, M. E. "The Effects of Progressive Resistance Training on Bone Density: A Review." *Med Sci Sports Exerc* 31:1(1999):25–30.
Lemole, G. M. *The Healing Diet.* New York: William Morrow, 2001.
Murakami, M., et al. "Effects of Epinephrine and Lactate on the Increase in Oxygen Consumption of Nonexercising Skeletal Muscle after Aerobic Exercise." *J Biomed Opt* 5:4(2000):406–410.

Nelson, M. E., et al. "Effects of High-Intensity Strength Training on Multiple Risk Factors for Osteoporotic Fractures: A Randomized, Controlled Trial." *JAMA* 272(1994):1909–1914.

Nelson, M. E., et al. "Analysis of Body-Composition Techniques and Models for Detecting Change in Soft Tissue with Strength Training." *Am J Clin Nutr* 63:5(1996):678–686.

Nelson, M. E., et al. "Hormone and Bone Mineral Status in Endurance-Trained and Sedentary Postmenopausal Women." *J Clin Endocrinol Metab* 66:5(1988):927–933.

Thomas, E. L., et al. "Preferential Loss of Visceral Fat Following Aerobic Exercise, Measured by Magnetic Resonance Imaging." *Lipids* 35:7(2000):769–776.

Van Aggel-Leijssen, D. P., Saris, W. H., Hul, G. B., and van Baak, M. A. "Short-Term Effects of Weight Loss with or without Low-Intensity Exercise Training on Fat Metabolism in Obese Men." *Am J Clin Nutr* 73:3(2001):523–531.

Sleep

Redwine, L., et al. "Effects of Sleep and Sleep Deprivation on Interleukin-6, Growth Hormone, Cortisol, and Melatonin Levels in Humans." *J Clin Endocrinol Metab* 85:10(2000):3597–3603.

Van Cauter, E., Leproult, R., and Plat, L. "Age-Related Changes in Slow Wave Sleep and REM Sleep and Relationship with Growth Hormone and Cortisol Levels in Healthy Men." *JAMA* 284:7(2000):879–881.

Walsleben, J. A. "Does Being Female Affect One's Sleep?" *J Womens Health Gender-Based Med* 8:5(1999):571–572.

http://www.sleepfoundation.org

Journaling

McGee-Cooper, A. "Time Management: Cashing in on Both Brains." *AORN J* 44:2(1986):178–183.

McGee-Cooper, A. "Shifting from High Stress to High Energy." *Imprint* 40:4(1993):69–71.

Pennebaker, J. W., and Seagal, J. D. "Forming a Story: The Health Benefits of Narrative." *J Clin Psychol* 55:10(1999):1243–1254.

CHAPTER 8

Mokdad, A. H., et al. "The Spread of the Obesity Epidemic in the United States, 1991–1998." *JAMA* 282(1999):1519–1522.

Must, A., et al. "The Disease Burden Associated with Overweight and Obesity." *JAMA* 282(1999):1523–1529.

"Now What? U.S. Study Says Margarine May Be Harmful." *New York Times* (October 1997).

"Update: Prevalence of Overweight among Children, Adolescents, and Adults—United States, 1988–1994." *MMWR* 46(1997):199–202.

CHAPTER 10

Finn, S. C. "Nutrition Communique: Helping Women Find Everyday Solutions." *J Womens Health Gender-Based Med* 9:9(2000):951–954.

U.S. Department of Agriculture, Agricultural Research Service. "Food and Nutrient Intakes by Individuals in the United States, by Sex and Age, 1994–1996," Nationwide Food Surveys, 1998.

"Women's Health Issues Survey." *Wirthlin Worldwide* (October 1999).

CHAPTER 11

Abraham, G. E. "The Calcium Controversy." *J Appl Nutr* 34(1982):69.

Abraham, G. E., and Grewal, H. "A Total Dietary Program Emphasizing Magnesium Instead of Calcium: Effect on the Mineral Density of Calcaneous Bone in Postmenopausal Women on Hormonal Therapy." *J Repr Med* 35(1990):503.

Abraham, G. E. "Nutritional Factors in the Etiology of the Premenstrual Tension Syndromes." *J Reprod Med* 28:7(1983):446–464.

Agostoni, C., et al. "Docosahexaenoic Acid Status and Developmental Quotient of Healthy Term Infants." *Lancet* 346(1995):638.

Aldercreitz, A. L., et al. "Dietary Phytoestrogen and the Menopause in Japan." *Lancet* 339(1992):1233.

Anderson, G. J., Connor, W. E., and Corliss, J. D. "Docosahexaenoic Acid Is the Preferred Dietary ω-3 Fatty Acid for the Development of the Brain and Retina." *Pediatr Res* 27(1990):89–97.

Barber, M. D., et al. "The Effect of an Oral Nutritional Supplement Enriched with Fish Oil on Weight Loss in Patients with Pancreatic Cancer." *Br J Cancer* 81:1(1999):80–86.

Bariscoe, A. M., and Ragen, C. "Relation of Magnesium and Calcium Metabolism in Man." *Am J Clin Nutr* 19(1966):296.

Berth-Jones, J., and Graham-Brown, R. A. "Placebo-Controlled Trial of Essential Fatty Acid Supplementation in Atopic Dermatitis." *Lancet* 341:8860(1993):1557–1560.

Berth-Jones, J., et al. "Evening Primrose Oil and Atopic Eczema." *Lancet* 345(1995):520.

Bhatty, R. S. "Nutrient Composition of Whole Flax Seed and Flax Seed Meal." In Cunnane S. C., Thompson, L. U. (eds.), *Flaxseed in Human Nutrition*. Chicago: AOCS Press, 1995, pp. 22–42.

Blaylock, R. *Excitotoxins: The Taste That Kills.* Santa Fe, NM: Health Press, 1997.

Booth, S. "Flaxseed Improves Blood Glucose Levels." *J Hum Nutr Diet* 13(2000):363–371.

Bordoni, A., et al. "Evening Primrose Oil in the Treatment of Children with Atopic Eczema." *Drugs Exp Clin Res* 14:4(1988):291–297.

Burgess, J. R., et al. "Long-Chain Polyunsaturated Fatty Acids in Children with Attention Deficit Hyperactivity Disorder." *Am J Clin Nutr* 71(2000):327–30S

Butchko, H., and Kotsonis, F. "Postmarketing Surveillance in the Food Industry: The Aspartame Case Study." *Nutr Toxicol* (1994):235–249.

Callender, K., et al. "A Double-Blind Trial of Evening Primrose Oil in the Premenstrual Syndrome." *Hum Psychopharmacol* 3(1988):57–61.

Cameron, A. T. "Iodine Prophylaxis and Endemic Goiter." *Can J Public Health* 21(1930):541–548.

Carter, J. F. "Sensory Evaluation of Flaxseed of Different Varieties." *Proc Flax Inst* 56(1996):201–203.

Cassidy, A. "Biological Effects of Plant Estrogens in Premenopausal Women." (Abstract A866) *Am Soc Exp Biol* (1993).

Cave, W. T., Jr. "Dietary Omega-3 Polyunsaturated Fats and Breast Cancer." *Nutrition* 12(Suppl, 1996):S39–S42.

Cherken, L. C. "Health Alert: Herbs and Drugs that Don't Mix." *Family Circle* (September 12, 2000).

Choi, D. E. "Glutamate Neurotoxicity and Diseases of the Nervous System." *Neuron* 1(1988):623–634.

Colquhoun, I., and Bunday, S. "A Lack of Essential Fatty Acids as a Possible Cause of Hyperactivity in Children." *Med Hypoth* 7(1981):673–679.

Connor, W. E., Lowensohn, R., and Hatcher, L. "Increased Docosahexaenoic Acid Levels in Human Newborn Infants by Administration of Sardines and Fish Oil during Pregnancy." *Lipids* 31(Suppl, 1996):S183–S187.

Connor, W. E. "Diabetes, Fish Oil, and Vascular Disease." *Ann Intern Med* 123:12(1995):950–952.

Connor, W. E. "Importance of ω-3 Fatty Acids in Health and Disease." *Am J Clin Nutr* 71(Suppl, 2000):171S–175S.

Coulombe, R. A., and Sharma, R. P. "Neurobiochemical Alterations Induced by the Artificial Sweetener Aspartame." *Toxicol Appl Pharmacol* 83(1986):79–85.

Dalderup, L. M. "The Role of Magnesium in Osteoporosis and Idiopathic Hypercalcaemia." *Voeding* 21(1960):424.

Davoli, E., et al. "Serum Methanol Concentrations in Rats and in Men after a Single Dose of Aspartame." *Food Chem Toxicol* 24:3 (1986):187–189.

Edwards, R., et al. "Omega-3 Polyunsaturated Fatty Acid Levels in the Diet and in Red Blood Cell Membranes of Depressed Patients." *J Affect Disord* 48(1998):149–155.

Flaten, H. "Fish-Oil Concentrate: Effects of Variables Related to Cardiovascular Disease." *Am J Clin Nutr* 52(1990):300–306.

Fotsis, T., et al. "Genistein, a Dietary Ingested Isoflavonoid, Inhibits Cell Proliferation and In Vitro Angiogenesis." *J Nutr* 125:3(Suppl, 1995):790S–797S.

Frahm, D. "For Stool Observation." *Health Quarterly* (Winter 1997):2–4.

Frank, B., et al. "A Prospective Study of Egg Consumption and Risk of Cardiovascular Disease in Men and Women." *JAMA* 281(1999): 1387.

Gittleman, A. L. *Why Am I Always So Tired?* New York: HarperSan Francisco, 1999.

Gittleman, A. L. *Guess What Came to Dinner?* New York: Avery, 2000.

Goh, Y. K., et al. "Effect of Omega-3 Fatty Acid on Plasma Lipids, Cholesterol, and Lipoprotein Fatty Acid Content in NIDDM Patients." *Diabetologia* 40(1997):45–52.

Goss, P. E, et al. *Effects of Dietary Flaxseed in Women with Cyclical Mastalgia.* Toronto: University Health Network/Princess Margaret Hospital, University of Toronto, 2000.

Harris, W. S. "Ω-3 Fatty Acids and Serum Lipoproteins: Human Studies." *Am J Clin Nutr* 65(Suppl, 1997):1645S–1654S.

Hederos, C. A., et al. "Epogam Evening Primrose Oil Treatment in Atopic Dermatitis and Asthma." *Arch Dis Child* 75:6(1996):494–497.

Heroux, O., Peter, D., and Heggteveit, H. A. "Long-Term Effect of Suboptimal Dietary Magnesium." *J Nutr* 107(1977):1640.

Hibbelin, J. R. "Fish Consumption and Major Depression (Letter)." *Lancet* 351(1998):1213.

Hibbelin, J. R., and Salem, N. "Dietary Polyunsaturated Fatty Acids and Depression: When Cholesterol Does Not Satisfy." *Am J Clin Nutr* 62(1995):1–9.

Holt, S. "Phytoestrogens for a Healthier Menopause." *Altern Complement Ther* 3:3(1997):187–193.

Horrobin, D. F. "Gamma Linolenic Acid." *Rev Contem Pharmacol* 1(1990):1–45.

Horrobin, D. F. "The Effects of Gamma Linolenic Acid on Breast Pain and Diabetic Neuropathy: Possible Non-Eicosanoid Mechanisms." *Prostaglandins Leukotrienes Essential Fatty Acids* 48(1993):101–104.

Hu, F. B. "A Prospective Study of Egg Consumption and Risk of Cardiovascular Disease in Men and Women." *JAMA* 281:15(1999):1387–1394.

Kahoo, S. K., et al. "Evening Primrose Oil and Treatment of Premenstrual Syndrome." *Med J Aust* 153(1990):192–198.

Knight, D. C., and Eden, J. A. "A Review of the Clinical Effects of Phytoestrogens." *Obstet Gynecol* 87(1996):897–904.

Kremer, J. M. "Ω-3 Fatty Acid Supplements in Rheumatoid Arthritis." *Am J Clin Nutr* 71(Suppl, 2000):349S–351S.

Kremer, J. M., et al. "Fish-Oil Fatty Acid Supplementation in Active Rheumatoid Arthritis: A Double-Blinded, Controlled, Crossover Study." *Ann Intern Med* 106(1987):497–503.

Levanthal, L. J., et al. "Treatment of Rheumatoid Arthritis with Gamma-Linolenic Acid." *Ann Intern Med* 1:9(1993):867–873.

Luo, J., et al. "Moderate Intake of ω-3 Fatty Acids for 2 Months Has No Detrimental Effect on Glucose Metabolism and Could Ameliorate the Lipid Profile in Type 2 Diabetic Men." *Diabetes Care* 21(1998):717–724.

McManus, R. M., et al. "A Comparison of the Effects of ω-3 Fatty Acids From Linseed Oil and Fish Oil in Well-Controlled Type II Diabetes." *Diabetes Care* 19(1996):463–467.

"Magnesium Deficiency in Alcoholism: Possible Contribution to Osteoporosis and Cardiovascular Disease in Alcoholics." *Alcoholism Clin Exp Res* 18:5(1994):1076–1082.

Makrides, M., Neumann, M. A., and Gibson, R. A. "Is Dietary Docosahexaenoic Acid Essential for Term Infants?" *Lipids* 31(1996):115–119.

Medalle, R., Waterhouse, C., and Hahn, T. J. "Vitamin D Resistance in Magnesium Deficiency." *Am J Clin Nutr* 29(1976):858.

Melis, M. S. "Stevia Dilates Vessels, Causing Lowered Blood Pressure and Increased Urine Flow When Given Over Long Periods." *J Ethnopharmacol* 47:3(1995):129–134.

Mitchell, E., et al. "Clinical Characteristics and Serum Essential Fatty Acid Levels in Hyperactive Children." *Clin Pediatr* 26(1987):406–411.

Mitchell, M. L., and O'Rourke, M. E. "Response of the Thyroid Gland to Thiocyanate and Thyrotropin." *J Clin Endocrinol* 20(1960):47–56.

Morton, M. S. "Determination of Lignans and Isoflavones in Human Female Plasma Following Dietary Supplementation." *J Endocrinol* 142(1994):251–259.

Moser, R. H. "Aspartame and Memory Loss." *JAMA* 272:19(1994):1543.

Olney, J. W. "Brain Lesions, Obesity, and Other Disturbances in Mice Treated with Monosodium Glutamate." *Science* 165(1969):719–721.

Olney, J. W. "Excitoxins and Neurological Diseases." In *Proceedings of the International College of Neuropathologists*, Kyoto, Japan, 1990.

Oomah, B. D., Mazza, G., and Kenaschuk, E. O. "Cyanogenic Compounds in Flaxseed." *J Agri Food Chem* 40(1992):1346–1348.

Reisbick, S., et al. "Home Cage Behavior of Rhesus Monkeys with Long-Term Deficiency of Omega-3 Fatty Acids." *Physiol Behav* 55(1994):231–239.

Roberts, H. J. "Reactions Attributed to Aspartame-Containing Products: 551 Cases." *J Appl Nutr* 40(1988):85–94.

Salachas, A., et al. "Effects of Low-Dose Fish Oil Concentrate on Angina, Exercise Tolerance Time, Serum Triglycerides, and Platelet Function." *Angiology* 45(1994):1023–1031.

Sojka, J. E., and Weaver, C. M. "Magnesium Supplementation and Osteoporosis." *Nutr Rev* 53(1995):71.

Stellman, F., and Garfinkel, L. "A Short Report: Artificial Sweetener Use and Weight Changes in Women." *Prevent Med* 15(1986):195–202.

Stevens, L. J., et al. "Essential Fatty Acid Metabolism in Boys with Attention-Deficit Hyperactivity Disorder." *Am J Clin Nutr* 62:4(1995):761–768.

Stevens, L. J., et al. "Omega-3 Fatty Acids in Boys with Behavior, Learning, and Health Problems." *Physiol Behav* 59:4–5(1996):915-920.

Tate, G., et al. "Suppression of Acute and Chronic Inflammation by Dietary Gamma Linolenic Acid." *J Rheumatol* 16(1989):729–734.

Tham, D. M. "Clinical Review 97: Potential Health Benefits of Dietary Phytoestrogens: A Review of the Clinical, Epidemiological, and Mechanistic Evidence." *J Clin Endocrinol Metabol* 83(1998):2223–2235.

Toft, I., et al. "Effects of ω-3 Polyunsaturated Fatty Acids on Glucose Homeostasis and Blood Pressure in Essential Hypertension." *Ann Intern Med* 123:12(1995):911–918.

"Turn Back the Clock with Nature's Fountain of Youth," *Health Sci Inst* 5:6(2000):1–5.

Uauy-Dagach, R., and Valenzuela, A. "Marine Oils: The Health Benefits of ω-3 Fatty Acids." *Nutr Rev* 54(1996):S102–S108.

Von Schacky, C., et al. "The Effect of Dietary Omega-3 Fatty Acids on Coronary Atherosclerosis." *Ann Intern Med* 130(1999):554–562.

Appendix

FAT FLUSH JOURNAL

PHASE ________

MY PHASE___ GOAL ______________________________

____

MY PHASE___ REWARD ______________________________

TODAY'S DATE ______________________________

Meals, Beverages & Snacks

- UPON RISING ______________________________
- BEFORE BREAKFAST ______________________________
- BREAKFAST ______________________________
- MIDMORNING SNACK ______________________________
- BEFORE LUNCH ______________________________
- LUNCH ______________________________

  ____

  ____

  ____

  ____
- MIDAFTERNOON SNACK ______________________________
- 4 P.M. SNACK ______________________________
- BEFORE DINNER ______________________________

©2002 Ann Louise Gittleman.

- DINNER
- MIDEVENING

Supplements

Measurements

- BUST/CHEST
- WAIST
- HIPS
- THIGHS

FOOD FOR THOUGHT

HEALTH & WELLNESS NOTES

©2002 Ann Louise Gittleman.

EXERCISE

SLEEP TIME

REFLECTIONS

DAILY ACKNOWLEDGMENT

©2002 Ann Louise Gittleman.

Index

About the Author

Top nutritionist Ann Louise Gittleman, M.S., C.N.S., is one of the most respected and dynamic nutritionsts in America today. She is recognized as an international authority on women's health and beauty having authored nearly twenty highly acclaimed books, including *Beyond Pritikin, The Living Beauty Detox*, and *Eat Fat, Lose Weight*. She is sits on the board of several nutritional foundations and is in demand as a guest on radio and television.

If you would like to be added to Ann Louise's mailing list or wish to contact her to arrange for a personal consultation or professional speaking engagement, she can be reached at **www.annlouise.com.**